Understanding Health System Change

Local Markets, National Trends

Understanding Health System Change

Local Markets, National Trends

Edited by Paul B. Ginsburg and Cara S. Lesser
Center for Studying Health System Change

Health Administration Press, Chicago, Illinois
Academy for Health Services Research and Health Policy, Washington, D.C.

05 04 03 02 01   5 4 3 2 1

Library of Congress Cataloging-in-Publication Data

Understanding health system change: local markets, national trends/ edited by Paul Ginsburg and Cara Lesser.
    p. cm.
    Includes bibliographical references.
    ISBN 1-56793-155-3 (alk. paper)
    1. Medical care—United States. 2. Medical policy—United States. 3. Managed care plans (Medical care)—United States. 4. Public health—United States. I. Ginsburg, Paul B. II. Lesser, Cara.
    RA399.A3 U48 2001
    362.1'0973—dc21

2001024268
CIP

The paper used in this publication meets the minimum requirements of American National Standard for Information Sciences—Permanence of Paper for Printed Library Materials, ANSI Z39.48-1984. ∞ ™

Project manager/Editor: Jane Williams; Book design: Matt Avery

Health Administration Press
A division of the Foundation of the
    American College of Healthcare Executives
1 North Franklin Street, Suite 1700
Chicago, IL 60606-3491
(312) 424-2800

Academy for Health Services
    Research and Health Policy
1801 K Street, Suite 701-L
Washington, DC 20006
(202) 292-6700

Table of Contents

Acknowledgment

Although each chapter in this book was written by one or two authors, the site visit data collection that underlies this research was a team effort conducted by staff from the Center for Studying Health System Change (HSC), The Lewin Group, and academic consultants. We would like to thank all of the individuals who participated in this effort for their contributions to the research.

We would like to particularly thank Ray Baxter and Caroline Steinberg, from The Lewin Group, for their leadership, insight, and reflection, which helped shape this research. We would also like to thank Jon Christianson, from the University of Minnesota, and Lawrence Brown, from Columbia University. Both were integral members of the data collection and analysis efforts and provided invaluable input and guidance.

We are especially indebted to the many people in the 12 communities from which we collected data. These people took time from their busy schedules to share with us their insights into the changes occurring in their local healthcare systems. We are particularly grateful to the individuals in each community who reviewed our draft reports and provided important suggestions. We would thank them by name, but we are restricted by our promise of confidentiality.

Finally, we are very grateful to The Robert Wood Johnson Foundation for its support of HSC and for funding this research.

Paul B. Ginsburg and Cara S. Lesser

Introduction

Cara S. Lesser, M.P.P., and Paul B. Ginsburg, Ph.D.

The period between 1997 and 1999 marked an important turning point in the development of the U.S. healthcare system. In prior years, managed care enrollment had soared and dramatic changes were anticipated in the organization and financing of healthcare. Expectations grew that under continuing pressure to control costs consumers would move into increasingly tightly managed health insurance products and healthcare providers and health plans would migrate toward more integrated systems of care to manage these arrangements. Integration was seen to have the potential to improve the quality of care—through more prevention, better coordination, and the use of evidence-based medicine—and to reduce costs. In many communities, hospitals, physicians, and health plans embarked on a number of strategies—from mergers and acquisitions to entry into new lines of business—which all together promised significant reorganization of local healthcare systems. The march toward managed care was interrupted, however, by a virulent consumer backlash against managed care. As healthcare organizations scrambled to adjust to a changing set of market conditions, many local healthcare systems experienced significant upheaval and a distinct shift occurred in the direction of healthcare systems nationally.

Although related information abounds about isolated communities or organizations, little systematic information exists on how healthcare systems as a whole are changing across the United States. The Center for Studying Health System Change (HSC) designed the Community Tracking Study (CTS) specifically to fill this information gap, documenting market changes and reflecting on their implications for consumers and for public policy. This book presents analyses of that study's second round of site visits, which were conducted between 1998 and 1999.

Based on the belief that healthcare is essentially a local service exchanged in a series of local markets, the CTS focuses on a group of communities that were selected to be representative of the United States. This focus allows HSC to reflect on how the healthcare system is changing nationally, while acknowledging variations at the local level.

Unlike other studies that focus on markets considered to be leaders or on the cutting-edge, the CTS focuses on 12 communities or study sites that were selected randomly from a stratified sample of metropolitan statistical areas with a population of 200,000 or more (see Kemper et al. 1996 for more detail on sample selection). This selection process yielded a diverse sample of markets, representing all regions of the United States—from large metropolitan areas such as Boston and Miami to smaller cities such as Syracuse and Lansing. Table 1 provides a complete list of the 12 communities that participate in the study and highlights some of their key characteristics.

In addition, the selection process resulted in a sample of communities with different histories, cultures, and experiences with managed care. For example, at one extreme is Orange County, California—a community with extensive history of HMO enrollment and powerful independent physician organizations. At the other extreme is Greenville, South Carolina, where few independent physician organizations have emerged and where HMOs have seen little growth. The study also features communities such as Indianapolis and Cleveland, where local not-for-profit hospitals play a leading role and operate some of the leading local health plans, and communities such as Phoenix, Miami, and Orange County, where nationally owned for-profit health plans dominate the market.

Background

HSC visits each of the 12 communities every two years to gather data through in-person interviews. These interviews provide a window into how local healthcare systems are evolving, including an examination of the forces that drive change in specific communities, the ways a diverse set of organizations respond to these forces, and the implications of change for community residents.

HSC's first round of CTS site visits was conducted between May 1996 and April 1997. Four-person teams visited each community for three to four days to conduct semistructured interviews with a broad cross-section of local healthcare system leaders. Respondents included representatives of local health plans, hospitals, and physician organizations as well as key employers in the community and state and local health policymakers. For additional perspective on the local market, the teams also conducted interviews with academics, reporters, and other observers of the healthcare system. In order to validate the data, responses were "triangulated"—that is, respondents' reports about developments at his or her organization were compared to reports from those in organizations that are competitors, suppliers, or customers. A total of roughly 40 to 60 interviews were conducted in each site, depending on the size of the community.

Despite variations across communities, several common themes emerged from the first round of site visits. Rapid managed care growth was anticipated in all communities, leading to extensive organizational change as hospitals and physicians sought to establish mechanisms for accepting financial risk for the delivery of care and for making the care delivery process more efficient (Kohn 2000). Hospital mergers were observed in 10 of the 12 sites, and multiple mergers occurred in five communities. Physicians moved into a variety of new organizations, from physician-hospital organizations to independent practice associations, and, in some instances, sold their practices to physician practice management companies. Health plans were changing rapidly as well, as they aggressively pursued geographic expansion and consolidation and developed new products to capture greater market share (Grossman 2000). State policymakers scurried to establish new regulations that could keep pace with the evolving managed care marketplace, while at the same time attempting to shift more Medicaid enrollees into HMOs (Solomon 1998).

These trends raised a number of compelling questions for our second round of site visits, which were conducted between 1998 and 1999. In addition to tracking how healthcare systems continued to evolve, we focused our return visits on the following questions or issues:

- How are hospital mergers implemented, and what impact do they have on local communities? What services and facilities are consolidated in the course of a merger, and what are the implications of mergers for hospital prices, access to care, and for communities' healthcare costs?
- As managed care enrollment grows and health plans consolidate rapidly, how are local Blue Cross and Blue Shield plans faring? Are these traditional health insurers becoming anachronistic or will they adapt to the changing environment, and what effect will this outcome have for local communities?
- How are specialists faring under a system that increasingly attempts to control utilization and costs of specialty care? What strategies are they pursuing to protect themselves in the managed care marketplace, and

TABLE 1: KEY CHARACTERISTICS OF 12 STUDY SITES

	Boston	Cleveland	Greenville	Indianapolis	Lansing	Little Rock	Miami
Demographics							
MSA population, July 1, 1999[1]	4,409,572	2,221,181	929,565	1,536,665	450,789	579,795	2,175,634
Population change 1990-1999, percent change[2]	3%	1%	12%	11%	4%	8%	12%
Median family income[3]	$31,868.25	$26,839.90	$24,967.36	$27,995.55	$30,829.70	$28,549.56	$19,672.17
Percent of population in poverty[3]	10%*	13%	14%	11%*	11%*	12%	25%*
Percent of population aged 65 and over[3]	14%*	15%*	13%*	12%	10%	12%	15%*
Health Insurance Status							
Percent of population under age 65 with no health insurance[3]	8%*	9%*	13%	14%	8%*	15%	23%*
Percent of children (under age 18) with no health insurance[3]	3%*	6%*	9%	10%	4%*	12%	17%*
Percent of employees working for private firms that offer coverage[4]	88%*	90%*	88%	86%	85%	82%	77%*
Average monthly premium for self-only coverage under employer-sponsored insurance[4]	$198.02*	$162.72*	$157.52*	$178.16	$182.73	$157.79*	$160.89*
Health System Characteristics							
Staffed hospital beds per 1000[5]	2.72	3.60	2.79	3.34	2.15	5.04	3.62
Total physicians per 1000 population[6]	3.28	2.74	1.73	2.48	2.14	3.07	2.73
HMO penetration,1997, percentage[7]	46%	27%	8%	23%	41%	25%	64%
HMO penetration, 1999, percentage[8]	48%	29%	13%	23%	41%	28%	52%

* Site value is significantly different from the average for large metropolitan areas

1 U.S. Census, 1999
2 U.S. Census, 1990 and 1999
3 Household Survey, Community Tracking Study, 1998-1999
4 Robert Wood Johnson Foundation Employer Health Information Survey, 1997

5 AHA Annual Survey Database™ for Fiscal Year 1998. Health Forum LLC, an American Hospital Association Company, copyright 2000.
6 Area Resource File, 1998
7 InterStudy Competitive Edge 8.1, July 1997
8 InterStudy Competitive Edge 10.1, July 1999

TABLE 1 (continued)

	Newark	Orange Cty	Phoenix	Seattle	Syracuse	Avg. Metro Areas[1]
Demographics						
MSA population, July 1, 1999[2]	1,954,671	2,760,948	3,013,696	2,334,934	732,920	200,099,042
Population change 1990-1999, percent change[3]	2%	15%	35%	15%	-1%	9%
Median family income[4]	$32,889.77	$30,634.89	$29,134.72	$34,565.75	$24,618.67	$27,842.61
Percent of population in poverty[4]	10% *	11%	14%	10% *	14%	14%
Percent of population aged 65 and over[4]	14% *	11%	13% *	12%	14% *	11%
Health Insurance Status						
Percent of population under age 65 with no health insurance[4]	12% *	18% *	17%	9% *	10% *	15%
Percent of children (under age 18) with no health insurance[4]	8%	15%	16% *	5% *	4% *	11%
Percent of employees working for private firms that offer coverage[5]	84%	81%	86%	85%	83%	84%
Average monthly premium for self-only coverage under employer-sponsored insurance[5]	$197.74	$156.10 *	$151.21 *	$182.81	$162.66 *	$181.05
Health System Characteristics						
Staffed hospital beds per 1000[6]	3.83	2.08	2.16	1.60	2.87	2.81
Total physicians per 1000 population[7]	2.64	2.16	1.74	2.47	2.35	2.29
HMO penetration,1997, percentage[8]	17%	46%	34%	29%	19%	32%
HMO penetration, 1999, percentage[9]	25%	46%	34%	20%	21%	36%

* Site value is significantly different from the average for large metropolitan areas

1 Average for metropolitan areas with 200,000 persons or more

2 U.S. Census, 1999

3 U.S. Census, 1990 and 1999

4 Household Survey, Community Tracking Study, 1998-1999

5 Robert Wood Johnson Foundation Employer Health Information Survey, 1997

6 AHA Annual Survey Database™ for Fiscal Year 1998. Health Forum LLC, an American Hospital Association Company, copyright 2000.

7 Area Resource File, 1998

8 InterStudy Competitive Edge 8.1, July 1997

9 InterStudy Competitive Edge 10.1, July 1999

what impact are these strategies having on the shape and functioning of the local healthcare system?

- How are states progressing with their efforts to move increasing numbers of Medicaid beneficiaries into HMOs, and what are the implications of these developments for Medicaid recipients and traditional providers of care for the low-income and uninsured?
- What forces are driving the development of new managed care regulations, and what impact are they having on health plans, providers, and consumers in local markets?

Site visits were conducted in each of the 12 communities between June 1998 and February 1999 to gather data on these issues and to obtain a general update on how the communities' healthcare systems had changed since the first round of visits. As in the first visit, three- to four-person teams visited each community, conducting a total of 30 to 60 interviews per site. Special interview protocols were designed to address each of the study issues, and specific respondent types were identified to gather perspectives from key actors knowledgeable about these issues. In addition to people who are directly involved in the implementation of the specific developments of interest, several "vantage" respondents were interviewed in each site to provide additional perspective and to allow researchers to "triangulate" results.

Findings from the 1998-1999 Site Visits

This book presents the major findings from the 1998-1999 site visits. Part I—Market Developments Across Communities—focuses on the major cross-site findings from our second round of site visits. Part II—Community Reports—contains an update on the local healthcare system for each of our 12 study sites. These analyses capture the richness in variation of healthcare system change at the local level.

Part I: Market Developments Across Communities

Chapter 1 is an overview of the key developments that emerged between the first (1996 to 1997) and second (1998 to 1999) rounds of visits. It highlights how backlash against managed care and consumer demand for less-restrictive insurance products gained force during this period, resulting in slow growth in HMO enrollment and a general retreat from the tightly managed products that many had expected to flourish by this time. This shift triggered a number of developments, which are counter to what had been anticipated in local healthcare systems. Capitation arrangements did not become more prevalent as many had predicted, and organizations continued to move away from vertically integrated models, which combined health insurance with the delivery of care. New organizational arrangements that allow providers to accept risk stumbled badly, and many of them folded during this time. What remained, however, was extensive consolidation in both the health plan and hospital sectors and continued pursuit of broad geographic scope to gain market share and bargaining power relative to one another. As a result, local healthcare systems have evolved in a manner that is likely to make future efforts to control costs more difficult.

Chapter 2 presents findings from the study of hospital mergers and their implications for local communities. The study indicates that although extensive consolidation of ownership has occurred in many communities, hospital mergers have not resulted in dramatic reorganization of local healthcare delivery systems. Most mergers in the study took steps to consolidate "back-room" administrative functions such as purchasing and finance, but few consolidated clinical service or clinical capacity that would have more visible effects in the community. As a result, the efficiency gains from mergers have been more modest than some anticipated. Rather, it appears that mergers have been most successful in helping hospitals to consolidate their bargaining power with payers, allowing them to stave off further declines in reimbursement and helping them to negotiate better managed care contracts. While this outcome is positive for consumers interested in protecting services and jobs in their local communities, it poses potential negative effects for the prospects of controlling hospital costs in the future.

Chapter 3 looks inside the health insurance industry to explore how local Blue Cross and Blue Shield Plans are faring in the changing marketplace. The Blues hold a unique place in communities' healthcare systems. Together, the Blues provide coverage to one in four Americans, representing the largest private payer in the United States. In addition, these local not-for-profit organizations historically received special regulatory treatment in exchange for providing health insurance coverage to all, often at rates that did not take into account health status or risk factors. Today, however, most differential regulatory treatment has disappeared, and Blue Plans operate in an increasingly competitive marketplace dominated by managed care products and national for-profit firms. Nevertheless, the Blues continue to be uniquely positioned in the market relative to their competitors, especially as the pendulum swings back toward a fee-for-service PPO market. With their large local market share and longevity in local markets, the Blues yield considerable market clout with providers and are able to offer purchasers and consumers attractive features, including broad provider and product choice, access to a valued brand name and national network, stability, and local accountability.

The Blues today, however, are making strategic choices that diminish some of the benefits that consumers have traditionally enjoyed from them, as they strive to balance the pressures to enhance margins against the demands of being a good corporate citizen. In the face of increased competition, the Blues are engaging in a significant amount of consolidation and conversion activity, which will likely erode the stability and local accountability of Blue Plans, particularly as some of the Plans will become relatively indistinguishable from their for-profit national competitors. To date, regulators have focused on protecting local public assets when scrutinizing conversions and mergers of the Blues. The authors argue, however, that policymakers should consider uniform regulation across all health plans to the extent that they want to use regulatory approaches to ensure access to affordable health insurance and local health plan accountability.

Chapter 4 turns to another important component of the healthcare system: specialists. Specialists control a substantial portion of healthcare spending and have been an important target for managed care plans in their efforts to hold down costs. Moreover, the perceived oversupply of specialists in many communities places them in a weak bargaining position with payers. However, we found that specialists have developed a number of strategies that help bolster their positions relative to health plans. Through practice mergers or joining IPAs, specialists in many communities have increased their leverage in managed care negotiations. Some of these efforts have resulted in virtual monopolies among certain specialties in geographic submarkets, providing these physicians considerable leverage and limiting the health plans' ability to achieve cost control through discounts. Some specialists also have pursued joint ventures with local hospitals or national management companies in an effort to capture some of the facility fees for their procedures and offset discounts for professional services under managed care contract arrangements. This activity threatens the loss of some of hospitals' most lucrative services, which some speculate could destabilize hospitals in the future.

Chapter 5 examines the evolution of Medicaid managed care across our 12 study sites, from "embryonic" (Greenville and Little Rock); to "established" (Orange County and Phoenix); to "emerging" (Cleveland, Indianapolis, Lansing, and Syracuse); and to "evolving" (Boston, Miami, Northern New Jersey, and Seattle). Despite differences in their stage of development, states have encountered a number of similar obstacles to the simultaneous goals of reducing costs and enhancing access and quality, including difficulties with setting payment rates and reporting requirements, variable plan participation, and outreach and enrollment processes. Traditional safety net providers of care for the low-income and uninsured have had mixed experiences with Medicaid managed care, with some providers continuing to struggle in the face of competition for their traditional clientele even in the most "established" markets. Ultimately, the author concludes that the cost savings anticipated under managed care may prove elusive; if so, he states that "the initial intellectual public offerings that put Medicaid in the managed care business would seem to need fresh conceptual capital."

Chapter 6 discusses another way that policy has shaped local healthcare systems: through increased managed care regulation. Capitalizing on the intense negative public opinion fostered largely by the media, physicians were identified as the prime movers for managed care regulation in the 12 study sites. Consumer advocates have weighed in as well, as have politicians who found that they could win political "mileage" on this hot-button issue from voters. In light of both real and anticipated new regulation, health plans have implemented new grievance procedures, eliminated gatekeeping requirements, and acquiesced to a number of patient-protection measures. Though observers may dismiss these developments as too little too late or too much too soon, the author argues that the subtle interplay of regulator and health plan interactions have produced meaningful results that can both protect consumer interests and preserve the managed care industry.

Part II: Community Reports

The Community Reports describe changes in individual local healthcare systems, highlighting key developments in our 12 study sites between the first visit in 1996-1997 and the return visit in 1998-1999. Several unique stories unfolded in these markets. In Boston, the city's large academic medical centers completed a series of mergers that considerably strengthened their leverage in managed care negotiations. In contrast, providers in Orange County were in disarray, as two large national physician practice management companies (PPMCs) went bankrupt, disrupting the extensive managed care contracting relationships that had been established in that market.

In many communities, the effects of managed care were more muted than anticipated—while many expected extensive downsizing and closures to emerge in local markets, instead many actually experienced further expansions. In Little Rock, for example, both inpatient and outpatient capacity continued to expand despite existing excesses. Similarly, in Cleveland, hospitals expanded high-end medical services, such as cardiac and cancer care, to attract more referrals and strengthen their revenue base.

State and local health policy also left its mark on several communities. The Seattle market saw turmoil in the individual insurance market and public programs to provide health insurance coverage for the poor as a result of unexpected interactions between these initiatives. On a more positive note, in both Indianapolis and Lansing, providers and policymakers were collaborating to develop new local programs to expand access to care for the uninsured using a managed care model.

These communities' healthcare systems continue to evolve—often in ways quite different from what local and national market observers expect. Updates from the third round of CTS site visits conducted in 2000 and 2001 are available on our web site (www.hschange.org).

Implications

This book provides insights into how local healthcare systems are changing and the issues that confront policymakers who seek to enhance access to, control costs of, and improve quality in the U.S. healthcare system. As our CTS continues with its current third round of site visits, we find that many of the trends identified in this book are continuing today. Early results suggest that local healthcare systems continue to move away from tightly managed health insurance products to the point where the long-term viability of traditional HMOs has been called into question in markets where they were once expected to flourish. At the same time, continued consolidation in local markets has helped organizations to develop greater leverage in negotiation with payers. Premiums have risen considerably, and providers have successfully begun to secure better contracting terms with health plans. As our analyses of our second visits suggest, these trends pose serious threats to the cost-control initiatives of the early 1990s. However, as costs begin to increase again, and the booming economy takes a turn, a change in direction is likely in the future. The key question to track will be how healthcare systems respond to renewed pressures to control costs at a time when the promise of managed care has come under siege.

PART ONE

*Market Developments
Across Communities*

CHAPTER 1

Retreat from Managed Care: How Local Healthcare Systems Changed, 1997-1999

Cara S. Lesser, M.P.P., and Paul B. Ginsburg, Ph.D.

Introduction

At the time of HSC's first round of site visits in 1996 to 1997, pressures for looser forms of managed care had already been noted. A very rapid shift toward managed care enrollment had led to demands from employees for less-restrictive forms of managed care (Christianson 1998). Policymakers were aggressively pursuing managed care enrollment for Medicaid and Medicare beneficiaries, while establishing a number of regulations aimed at limiting what many viewed as the more restrictive practices of managed care plans (Solomon 1998).

Health plans and providers were actively positioning themselves in response to these divergent demands. Health plans' strategies centered on consolidation and geographic expansion, aggressive pricing to expand market share, and development of less-restrictive managed care products (Grossman 2000). Providers were making efforts to consolidate and develop new organizational arrangements and partnerships for contracting with managed care organizations (Kohn 2000). Both health plans and

This chapter was adapted, with permission from Project Hope, from the original article published in *Health Affairs* (Nov/Dec 2000): "Update on the Nation's Health Care System: Results from Tracking Change in 12 Communities, 1997-1999," by Cara S. Lesser and Paul B. Ginsburg.

The authors are grateful to Joy Grossman, Peter Kemper, Ray Baxter, Caroline Steinberg, and an anonymous referee from *Health Affairs* for providing valuable comments to this chapter.

providers also experimented with ways to make care delivery more efficient and to reap the benefits of these savings, with innovative payment arrangements and mechanisms for monitoring and reporting on practice patterns (Kohn 2000).

This chapter examines how communities' healthcare systems have evolved over the two years since then. Following a brief review of our site visit methodology, this chapter discusses the intensification of consumer backlash against managed care and its effect on product types and payment arrangements. Against this backdrop, we describe major changes in the strategies of healthcare organizations, including the move away from vertical integration and intermediary organizations toward a competitive dynamic that emphasizes horizontal consolidation and the pursuit of regional scope. Our discussion concentrates on the implications of these changes for consumers' access to care and the efficiency of the system.

Findings

Our findings are best understood through a framework of the demand (consumers and purchasers) and supply (providers and health plans) sides of a market. During this period a demand-side trend toward looser forms of managed care accelerated (unexpectedly to some respondents) and caused tremendous turmoil on the supply side, as strategies that had been conceived in an era in which highly-integrated managed care was seen as the wave of the future unraveled. One important exception was health plan and provider strategies of horizontal consolidation, which became increasingly emphasized.

Backlash and Increased Demand for More Loosely Managed Products

While consumers have voiced concern about managed care for several years (Blendon et al. 1998), the backlash against managed care intensified between 1997 and 1999 and began to have visible effects on local markets. Backed by employers and state legislative efforts, consumer demand for less-restrictive products gained force during this period and was reflected in changes in enrollment patterns, product offerings, and health plan policies. In contrast to widespread prior expectations about how healthcare markets would evolve, this period was noted for slow HMO growth and a general retreat from highly managed products.

Strong economic growth and tight labor markets contributed to an environment of heightened consumer expectations and increased willingness on the part of employers to accommodate employee preferences for more loosely managed health insurance products (Gabel 1997; Grossman 2000;

Jensen et al. 1997; Robinson 1999). As in the first round of site visits, employers noted a continued emphasis on offering products with broad networks, out-of-network coverage, and less-restrictive access to care (Christianson 1998; Grossman 2000). This stance was particularly noteworthy in high-tech labor markets such as Boston and Seattle, where employers expressed reluctance to promote more restrictive insurance products or limit employees' choice of providers out of concern that these actions would put them at a disadvantage in competing for skilled labor.

Market demand for more loosely managed health insurance products has been bolstered by the flurry of recent state legislative activity to regulate managed care. Between 1997 and 1999, new state regulations designed to restrict managed care were established in all 12 of our study sites, regardless of the level of HMO penetration in the community or the presence of existing legislation in the state.[1] The new regulations, commonly enacted under the auspices of an omnibus "health care quality act" or "patient protection act," focused on three primary areas: mandated benefits, grievance procedures, and consumer protections, with many having provisions in two or three areas (see Table 1.1).

Some of these new regulations, such as those that require health plans to offer certain types of products or establish requirements regarding plan operations, have had direct effects on the structure and types of the products offered in these markets. However, the most significant effect of the new managed care regulations was indirect in their contribution to the overall climate, favoring less restrictive management of care. Slower-than-expected growth in HMO enrollment[2] was noted by respondents across all of our study sites, despite at least some increase since 1996 to 1997 in most sites (see Table 1.2). The average large metropolitan area experienced only a 7-percentage point increase in HMO enrollment between 1996 and 1998. Even markets that exceeded this average saw far less rapid growth than had been anticipated. For example, in Seattle, where HMO enrollment increased by 10 percentage points, an even greater boost was expected. The community's largest employer, Boeing, recently had implemented an aggressive initiative to encourage employees to enroll in HMOs, and many expected other local employers to follow suit. However, other employers did not follow Boeing's lead, and the extensive marketwide shift to HMOs many had anticipated did not occur.

Our recent site visits also reinforced the finding from the previous round that enrollees in preferred provider organizations (PPOs)[3] appear unlikely to convert into HMO products as many predicted (Grossman 2000; Christianson 1998). For example, Greenville saw virtually no increase in HMO penetration over the two-year period despite some expectations that the community's large PPO enrollment would begin to

TABLE 1.1: SUMMARY OF SELECTED MANAGED CARE REGULATIONS
ENACTED SINCE ROUND 1 SITE VISITS *(current as of May 31, 1999)*

Study Site	Grievance Procedures or Review Processes	Consumer Protection	Mandated Benefits
Boston	Yes*	No	No
Cleveland	Yes	Yes	Yes
Greenville	No	Yes	Yes
Indianapolis	Yes	Yes	Yes
Lansing	Yes	Yes	Yes
Little Rock†	Yes	Yes	Yes
Miami	Yes	Yes	Yes
Northern New Jersey‡	Yes	Yes	Yes
Orange County	Yes	Yes	Yes
Phoenix	Yes	No	Yes
Seattle	No	Yes	No
Syracuse	Yes	Yes	Yes
Total Number of Sites	10	10	10

* Passed via governor's executive order.
† The Assembly was not in session at the time of the Round 2 visit. Developments
   represent what happened during and immediately after the Round 1 site visit in 1996.
‡ Northern New Jersey is defined by the Newark primary metropolitan statistical area
   (PMSA) and includes Sussex, Warren, Morris, Essex, and Union counties.

Note: Data for this chart are drawn from the National Conference of State Legislatures'
Health Policy Tracking Service and were confirmed during our site visits and follow-up
phone interviews. The categories are defined to include the following:

- *Grievance procedures or review processes:* Requirements pertaining to external review and
   grievance processes, mandated timeframe for internal reviews of appeals, and other
   requirements concerning HMO internal review procedures and arbitration decisions.
- *Consumer protections:* Requirements pertaining to plan product offerings and product
   design (such as mandatory POS option, restrictions on "gag clauses," adequate choice of
   providers, access to nonformulary prescription drugs, and ability to seek out-of-network
   care for limited price differential); disclosure of information regarding provider network
   and plan performance; liability requirements regarding risk-based capital or other financial
   solvency standards; and any-willing-provider provisions.
- *Mandated benefits:* Requirements to cover certain services according to a set standard,
   such as prudent layperson standard for emergency room services or 48-hour hospital
   stays for deliveries, and requirements to allow direct access to certain providers, such as
   OB/GYNs.

TABLE 1.2: HMO PENETRATION 1996 TO 1998

Study Site	January 1996*	January 1998†	Change in Percentage Points 1996 to 1998
Boston‡	35%	49%	14
Cleveland	18	27	9
Greenville	10	10	0
Indianapolis	17	23	6
Lansing	32	41	9
Little Rock	33	27	-6
Miami	46	64	18
Northern New Jersey§	21	24	3
Orange County	41‖	46	5
Phoenix	27	34	7
Seattle	19	29	10
Syracuse	14	20	6
Metropolitan Area >200,000	27%	34%	7%
US (metro and nonmetro)	18%	33%	15%

* InterStudy Competitive Edge Regional Market Analysis, 6.2, September 1996.

† InterStudy Competitive Edge Regional Market Analysis, 8.2, December 1998.

‡ The Boston Community Tracking Study site varies slightly from the MSA definition. Estimates for the population HMO enrollment have been adjusted to reflect this variation.

§ Northern New Jersey is defined by the Newark primary metropolitan statistical area (PMSA) and includes Sussex, Warren, Morris, Essex and Union counties.

‖ January 1996 InterStudy data on Orange County is not available; instead, we have used InterStudy Competitive Edge Regional Market Analysis, 7.1, June 1997.

Note: There was a change in InterStudy methodology for calculating market share during this period, which may affect the numbers listed here.

transition into more restrictive products. Indeed, in many markets, PPO enrollment continued to grow rapidly; respondents now reject the notion that this is a transitional product that will lead to HMO enrollment.

Instead, this period was marked by stepped-up efforts on the part of health plans to reconfigure their HMO products to make them less restrictive. Two years earlier, health plans across our study sites were already responding to purchaser demands for provider choice and improved access to specialists by expanding networks of their existing products, easing gatekeeping restrictions and offering "open access" and point-of-service (POS) options in their HMO product lines (Grossman 2000). But between 1996 to 1997 and 1998 to 1999, these efforts to loosen up HMOs had become even more pronounced.

Across sites, respondents reported that broad and inclusive provider networks have become the norm among health plans. Gatekeeping restrictions that require patients to obtain approval from a primary care physician for access to certain services or referrals have become less popular. At the same time, gains in market share were often attributed to strong POS products, which provide for out-of-network coverage, and "open-access" products, which allow enrollees to have direct access to certain specialists within a closed panel of providers. United Healthcare's "open access" product was noted in several sites as a popular product and important to helping the plan build market share. For example, in Seattle, respondents attribute United's success with growing the small local market share, which it acquired from its merger with Travelers, largely to this product.

In addition, in several sites, health plans made more behind-the-scenes changes in how they manage care, revamping their approaches to appeals, the services they cover, and how they monitor utilization. Some of these changes were directly related to new regulations as health plans have had to expand their benefits or adopt new grievance procedures to comply with current law. In other cases, however, health plans made changes proactively in response to environmental pressure for less-restrictive products and/or in anticipation of new regulations. For example, in a number of communities, market respondents noted that plans had become increasingly willing to reverse decisions to deny care when challenged through an appeals process. Respondents viewed these developments as the health plans' efforts to demonstrate consumer responsiveness, while moving away from care management techniques that have not proved cost effective.

Slow Growth of Capitation

As health plans moved toward more loosely managed products, growth in the use of capitation to pay providers stagnated in most markets, and a number of communities experienced significant disruption from failures of organizations that had accepted extensive capitated risk. At the time of the first site visit, our survey data indicated that capitation accounted for 16 percent of physicians' total practice revenue, with substantial variation across sites. The most common type of capitation involved providers accepting risk for the services they deliver themselves, such as primary care physicians accepting capitated payment for primary care services. Global capitation arrangements—in which providers or provider-contracting intermediaries accept risk for a wide array of services such as physician, hospital, and ancillary services—were infrequent, with the exception of Orange County and Indianapolis (Kohn 2000). Regardless of this low baseline, however, there was widespread anticipation that capitation arrangements, and global capitation arrangements in particular, would flourish quite rapidly. Providers were actively positioning themselves for this growth in the hopes of capturing savings from the more-efficient delivery of care (Kohn 2000).

By 1998 to 1999, however, capitation arrangements did not proliferate as anticipated, and in several communities, health plans and providers experienced serious setbacks as a result of experiments with global capitation in particular. In markets such as Indianapolis, Phoenix, Miami, and Northern New Jersey, physicians and hospitals collaborated to establish new contracting vehicles to secure contracts with health plans that would pay for a broad range of services on the basis of capitation; but these contracts failed to materialize.

Provider respondents contended that health plans were reluctant to delegate financial risk and associated responsibility for care management to a coordinated physician-hospital organization that could exert significant market power. Health plan respondents, in turn, contended that their reluctance to enter into broad-scale capitation arrangements stemmed from concerns about the adequacy of provider organizations' infrastructure to manage financial risk and utilization. In addition, the increased emphasis on more loosely managed products made the delegation of substantial levels of risk more difficult and hindered its growth.

Meanwhile, in markets where extensive capitation arrangements had been established, physician organizations encountered serious difficulties, leading providers to back away from these arrangements as well. In Orange County, many providers had begun to participate in global capitation arrangements, thanks in part to the rapid growth of national PPMCs that aggressively pursued these contracts in key markets such as southern California. However, these organizations struggled with higher-than-expected cost increases from factors that they believed to be outside of their control, such as increased pharmaceutical costs and expansions of mandated benefits.

Orange County providers also reported difficulty managing the less-restrictive products that were gaining popularity among consumers. For example, under POS products, plans typically reduced providers' capitation rates to account for enrollees' use of out-of-network providers. However, providers contended that patients' out-of-network use was adding onto, rather than substituting for, in-network use. As a result, providers reported that capitation rates under POS products were particularly inadequate.

Although both health plans and providers began to approach capitation with greater caution, neither abandoned this payment model altogether. Rather, in many markets, providers and plans continued to experiment with ways to fine tune these arrangements in order to control costs and offer opportunity for both parties to benefit from the potential savings from increased efficiency in care delivery. For example, in Orange County and Indianapolis, many providers insisted that health plans retain some level of financial responsibility for difficult-to-control components such as pharmacy costs. Some isolated cases also emerged where providers and plans were experimenting with "contact capitation," which attempts to adapt risk arrangements to the demands for direct access to specialists and out-of-network utilization.

Moreover, in some of the communities, providers and health plans remained committed to pursuing global capitation and maintained expectations for its growth. In Boston, systems led by academic medical centers focused greater attention on their global risk contracts, even though these arrangements remained a relatively small share of their business and reportedly had not been profitable to date. Nevertheless, with the expectation that these contracts would grow, they invested heavily in the infrastructure needed to support them and continued to push health plans to entrust them with more responsibility for care management. Even Orange County, where the greatest disruption from failed global capitation arrangements occurred, showed no indication that the market was moving away from this model. Instead, the market experienced increased attention to regulatory reforms and independent industry initiatives to develop better ways to structure and oversee these arrangements, signaling their expected staying power in the market.

Vertical Disintegration

As markets retreated from highly managed health insurance products and stumbled with capitated payment arrangements, they also experienced a continued trend away from the vertically integrated organizational models, which only a few years ago were envisioned as the future of healthcare delivery. At the time of the first round of site visits, and even in the preceding pilot study site visits in 1995, the evidence was clear that organizations were moving away from combining insurer and provider functions under owned and exclusive arrangements (Grossman 2000). At the time of our 1996 to 1997 visits, long-standing staff and group model HMOs, such as Harvard Pilgrim Health Care in Boston and Intergroup-Foundation

Healthcare in Phoenix, had recently spun off their provider capacity, while a number of providers had opted to sell off their health plan subsidiaries (Grossman 2000). Two years later, few vertically integrated models remain in the communities we track.

During this period, abandonment of vertical integration strategies was seen most markedly among providers. Plans' efforts to unwind owned and exclusive arrangements appear to have occurred primarily in earlier years, as they attempted to respond to purchaser demand for broad networks and redress the productivity losses associated with salaried physicians (Grossman 2000; Robinson 1999). Over the past two years, however, providers' divestitures of health plans accelerated. In Seattle, three provider organizations sold off their health plans, including the prestigious multispecialty group Virginia Mason Medical Center, which sold its plan to Aetna U.S. Healthcare. Similarly, in Phoenix the area's largest hospital system, Samaritan Health System, sold its sizable commercial and Medicaid plans to United Healthcare.

Providers abandoned their vertical integration strategies for the same reasons noted among plans in the previous round of site visits (Grossman 2000). Respondents contended that significant investment of energy and capital was necessary to develop these new lines of business and these efforts distracted them from their core activities. Cultural differences between staff of health plan and provider lines of business also were more of an obstacle than anticipated. At the same time, soft premium rates dampened profitability in the health plan line of business and may have hastened providers' decision to exit. Some of the plans sold had been reasonably successful, but the capital that could be raised by selling them often was needed in the core hospital operation.

Consistent with these divestitures, providers made no new efforts to establish their own health plans. This finding stands in contrast to expectations two years earlier that these arrangements would flourish under the new option for provider-sponsored organizations (PSOs) to contract directly with the federal government for Medicare risk business.

Remaining instances in which providers have continued to operate their own plans tend to be in markets with highly concentrated provider systems, such as Lansing, Syracuse, and Indianapolis. Many traditional safety net providers also have maintained health plans to serve the Medicaid managed care population.

Demise of Provider Intermediary Organizations

At the time of our first round of site visits, local healthcare markets were experiencing the rapid growth of new organizations seeking to serve as contracting intermediaries between providers and plans; but within two years, many of these experimental models failed. Across all of the study sites, providers were actively forming independent practice associations (IPAs), physician-hospital organizations (PHOs), and management services organizations (MSOs) to enable them to accept capitated contracts from health plans or to blunt downward pressure on payment rates (Kohn 2000). At the same time, PPMCs were just beginning to emerge, purchasing physician practices in key markets with the promise of providing management services, gleaning efficiencies from economies of scope and scale, and bargaining with health plans from a stronger position. By the time of our second round of site visits, many of these new organizations had stumbled badly.

Unrealized expectations concerning risk contracting was commonly cited as a factor in the demise of these organizations. However, as noted previously, this story cut two ways. In some communities, such as Miami and Northern New Jersey, PHOs and IPAs struggled in the absence of risk contracts, which they had been created to manage. But in communities such as Orange County, where risk contracting was well established, several organizations—most prominently PPMCs—suffered from their inability to keep costs below the capitation rates they had negotiated.

Provider intermediary organizations faced internal management problems as well. PHOs, which commonly have been led by hospital administrators, often could not garner the trust of physicians; respondents noted that physicians often feel that PHOs negotiate health plan contracts that are good deals for the hospital but not for physicians. This tension contributed to the demise of several PHOs and has led toward more arms-length relationships between hospitals and physicians elsewhere.

Perhaps most disconcerting from the perspective of many stakeholders was the lack of progress in developing the infrastructure necessary to manage financial risk and to streamline and improve clinical care delivery. PPMCs, in particular, touted these advances as the great promise of their organizational model. However, respondents contended that PPMCs placed too much attention on the acquisition of practices at the expense of investing in these activities. Some suggest that the organizations lost the leadership resources essential to making these advances when key physicians defected from the organizations due to management disputes or sudden wealth brought on by the sale of their practices. Others noted that the transition to compensation via salary diminished physicians' incentives to push for such advances. Finally, some argue that PPMCs simply did not have the time needed to achieve these far-reaching goals in an environment of deteriorating physician bargaining power with health plans and pressure from Wall Street investors for quick success. Ultimately, market observers contended that these organizations got too big, too fast, adding costly and often redundant layers of overhead and providing little value in return.

The downfall of the PPMCs, in particular, caused considerable upheaval in communities where they had made significant inroads and had begun to reshape provider-plan relationships. The greatest effect was observed in Orange County, where two PPMCs—MedPartners and FPA Medical Management, Inc.—and their affiliated contracting entities included a significant portion of the market's physicians and acted as a critical component of health plans' contracting arrangements. Their unanticipated bankruptcies not only rendered worthless the stock these physicians received in exchange for the assets of their practices but also left numerous physicians practices that were owned by the PPMCs without a vehicle for contracting with health plans. FPA also had been in Phoenix, and although it did not involve as many physicians, its bankruptcy had significant psychological impact on the market as it resulted in the dissolution of a long-respected local multispecialty group. Many respondents viewed the failure of PPMCs as a setback to physician-organization activity in general, even in markets where they had not secured an important role.

Hospitals, meanwhile, began to reassess their physician integration strategies. Several shut down their PHOs and, in some instances, reconstituted them as IPAs and MSOs that have lower overhead and provide more targeted services to physicians. In some cases, physicians rejected hospital-led organizations altogether in favor of physician-led organizations. For example, physician-led IPAs gained membership rapidly in Syracuse, Miami, and Phoenix.

In other communities, however, especially where the hospital market is highly concentrated, hospitals continue to play a leading role as intermediaries. In Boston, for example, its two major academic medical center systems—Partners HealthCare and CareGroup—have established provider networks with more than 3,500 and 3,000 physicians, respectively, and continue to act as the major unifying force for managed care contracting.

Horizontal Consolidation and Pursuit of Regional Scope

While provider intermediaries stumbled and healthcare organizations continued to move away from vertical integration, the emphasis on horizontal consolidation strategies and the pursuit of broad geographic scope continued during this period. As in previous years, most of this activity involved hospitals and health plans, with physician consolidation lagging considerably (Kohn 2000).

At the time of our first round of site visits, local health plans across our study sites were involved in mergers, acquisitions, and joint ventures to build enrollment, expand networks or product lines, and fend off competitors and potential outside entrants to the market. Much of this activity revolved around geographic expansion to respond to employer demand for broad geographic coverage and to pursue economies of scale to compete with national health plans (Grossman 2000). Similarly, hospitals were consolidating rapidly, with mergers recently announced or underway in 10 of the 12 sites. This activity focused largely on regional expansion as well, with the goal of enhancing hospitals' indispensability to health plans' networks and gaining economies of scale in response to the competitive threats posed by aggressive expansion of national hospital chains, especially Columbia/HCA (Kohn 2000).

Two years later, merger activity among hospitals slowed and was no longer driven by the threat of outside entry, which was pervasive two years earlier. The reversal of Columbia's aggressive acquisition strategy removed a key competitive pressure for hospitals in all sites. In some instances, however, Columbia's decision to exit certain markets produced further concentration of ownership as local systems acquired these holdings. This occurred in Cleveland, where Columbia's decision to sell off its 50 percent share of the Sisters of Charity system created an acquisition opportunity for University Hospitals Health System (UHHS). As a result of this and other recent consolidation, UHHS and the Cleveland Clinic Health System now control all but a handful of independent community hospitals in the market.

The extensive consolidation that had already occurred in communities also contributed to a slowdown of hospital merger activity. Indeed, by the time of the second round of visits, the hospital sector in most sites had become or was in the process of becoming largely concentrated in just two to four systems. While some markets historically have been concentrated, significant change occurred in many of our study sites over the past few years. Increased concentration was observed in markets of varying size, including large markets such as Boston and Miami; mid-size markets such as Cleveland and Indianapolis; and small metropolitan markets such as Lansing and Syracuse.

Despite increased concentration of ownership, however, limited consolidation of services or capacity has taken place. As in our first round of site visits, little evidence suggested that hospitals were making the "hard decisions" to close facilities, reduce beds, or eliminate duplicative services (Kohn 2000). Rather, the desire to maintain a full spectrum of services across a broad geographic area to attract managed care contracts and draw in referrals has worked against closing duplicative services in neighboring markets. Moreover, in some instances, these market conditions appeared to be creating incentives to expand existing services and excess capacity. For example, in Cleveland, the two major provider systems added services in suburban areas outside of their core markets. Similar expansions of services and capacity—largely outpatient but some inpatient—were observed in others markets such as Little Rock, Indianapolis, and Phoenix.

Hospitals' continuing emphasis on achieving broad regional scope came in part from health plans' parallel emphasis on consolidation and geographic expansion. Unlike in the hospital sector, national firms continued to play a leading role in health plan merger activity, with mergers and acquisitions among national plans producing greater market concentration and/or new entry in a number of our study sites. The most striking example was seen in Northern New Jersey, where the Aetna U.S. Healthcare merger—first with NYLCare and more recently with Prudential—consolidated more than 40 percent of local HMO market share with the plan. Though HMO enrollment still represented only a relatively small portion of the market (24 percent), Aetna's dominance in this segment of the market raised concern for many local respondents. In other communities, national plans' acquisition of local entities facilitated entry in the local market or expansion of market share. For example, Aetna's acquisition of the Virginia Mason Medical Center plan brought it back into the Seattle market, while in Phoenix, United's purchase of Samaritan Health System's two plans boosted it to become the second largest plan locally in terms of overall market share.

At the same time, the perceived and real threat of national firms' growing presence has led local plans to continue to pursue horizontal consolidation and geographic expansion during this period as well. For example, in Syracuse, the area's largest plan, Blue Cross and Blue Shield, of Central New York, now Excellus BlueCross BlueShield, gained significantly broader geographic reach as a result of its merger with Blues plans in neighboring Rochester and Utica. Another merger involving Syracuse- and Buffalo-based plans also created a new regional plan to compete in this area.

Local health plans also pursued regional scope by expanding into new geographic markets on their own. Extensive activity in this regard was observed in Northern New Jersey, where Blue Cross and Blue Shield of New Jersey began to expand into markets in neighboring states; Blues plans in New York, Pennsylvania, and Delaware, on the other hand, made forays into New Jersey.

However, for some plans, geographic expansion led to serious difficulty. The most salient example was seen in Boston, where Tufts Health Plan and Harvard Pilgrim Health Plan incurred substantial losses from operations in neighboring markets. These experiences suggest the possibility of dis-economies associated with horizontal consolidation and geographic expansion strategies, as have been noted among vertical integration strategies in recent research (Grossman 2000; Robinson 1999).

Despite continued consolidation among health plans, when one looks across all insurance products—from indemnity to HMOs—those markets defined as fragmented at the time of the first site visit (i.e., Miami, Northern New Jersey, and Phoenix) (Grossman 2000) remained so two years later. Although consolidation has produced fewer competitors in these markets, multiple plans remained, and market share was widely distributed among them. In addition, although national mergers led to entry and consolidation across several markets, local plans continued to maintain a leading position in most markets. Nonetheless, respondents viewed the growing presence and market share of national, for-profit firms as a continuing, and in some cases intensifying, threat to local plans in several study sites.

Conclusion: Implications for Consumers

The period between 1997 and 1999 marked a continuing movement away from the tightly managed products and the vertically integrated model, which many associate with managed care and expected local healthcare systems would evolve into over time. While these trends had been noted in previous years, during this period, these strategies stopped being perceived as a tactical retreat and became seen as a real change in direction. Rather than proceeding toward increasingly integrated provider and health plan functions and more restrictive provider networks, healthcare markets have been reverting to a more "traditional" organizational model, although with a much higher degree of horizontal consolidation and a much greater emphasis on geographic breadth and unfettered access. If a theory of market evolution were developed today, it likely would focus on the march toward increasing consolidation rather than the drive toward integration emphasized in earlier research (APM/University Health System Consortium 1995).

This shift has important implications for consumers. On the one hand, these changes have been responsive to consumer demand for unrestricted access to care and choice of providers. However, the way in which local markets are evolving threatens to jeopardize the cost control that has been achieved in recent years and to stunt the drive to produce further efficiencies necessary to maintain an affordable, accessible healthcare system.

Consolidation and geographic expansion have been pursued extensively, yet it appears that these strategies continue to be focused primarily on enhancing organizations' market power, often at the expense of opportunities to reduce costs. This dynamic, noted in our previous work, was seen most clearly during this period in the efforts of providers to expand regionally, where the quest for bargaining power was clearly more compelling than opportunities to rationalize duplicative services and excess capacity. The highly consolidated market structure that has emerged in communities' healthcare systems has created greater equilibrium among plans and major provider organizations, but it also leaves both parties in a stronger position to withstand pressure to control costs and become more efficient.

Both plans and providers continue to experience significant financial pressure from the demands of employers and shareholders and from cuts in Medicare reimbursement. Financial pressure on providers contributes to greater conflict between hospitals and physicians over a shrinking pie. But growing provider bargaining power appears to have slowed or stopped the trend toward greater price discounts, suggesting that cost-control gains may now plateau or begin to reverse.

With shrinking resources, and in the aftermath of many failed innovative organizational and payment arrangements, healthcare organizations appear increasingly wary of developing new and potentially risky ventures that promise to streamline the delivery of care. While many organizations continue to develop initiatives aimed at improving the quality of care and reducing unnecessary costs, great skepticism exists about the ability to produce significant efficiencies in the delivery of care, at least in the near term.

Developments in information technology and Internet-based solutions in particular present one potential exception. However, expectations of information technology transforming the delivery of care have met with disappointment for many years now. The decentralized nature of the Internet and, at least until recently, the ready availability of capital to finance Internet healthcare companies have lowered barriers to feasibility, but the success of these ventures remains to be seen.

Another significant development that could alter the current trajectory of change is a return to higher rates of increase in health insurance premiums. Although tight labor markets are delaying bold responses to higher premium increases on the part of employers currently, responses are probably only two years off. Once employers do respond, we expect more of an emphasis on patient cost sharing and financial incentives for employees to choose options involving more restrictive forms of managed care. In an environment in which managed care has become so stigmatized, consumers will be faced with the decision of assuming greater financial burden for unfettered access to care or pushing the industry and/or policymakers toward alternate solutions to contain costs and preserve access.

Notes

1. Boston was the only site where new legislation was not passed, although new regulations concerning grievance procedures and provider reimbursement were implemented through the governor's executive order in May 1998.
2. We define HMO products to include those in which individuals are provided healthcare services by a network of affiliated providers where services delivered by providers outside of the network are generally not covered, other than for some specialized services or in emergencies. To be consistent with the InterStudy data referred to in Table 1.2 and often cited by local respondents, we include enrollment in POS products as a form of HMO enrollment. POS products allow individuals to select in-network or out-of-network providers at the "point-of-service," usually with significant differences in coinsurance or deductibles. These products are sometimes referred to as "open-ended" HMOs or "triple option" plans.
3. PPOs are defined as products in which enrollees are given a financial incentive to use a "preferred" network of providers, usually through differences in coinsurance or deductibles.

CHAPTER 2

Hospital Mergers and Their Impact on Local Communities

Cara S. Lesser, M.P.P., and Linda R. Brewster, M.B.A.

Introduction

Mergers had become pervasive among hospitals by the mid-1990s, generating a great deal of speculation about the impact of these arrangements on local communities. More than 700 mergers and acquisitions were completed among hospitals between 1994 and 1997, involving roughly 300 hospitals each year (Irving Levin Associates 1999). HSC's first round of CTS site visits in 1996 to 1997 underscored the prevalence of this strategy: Hospital mergers were recently announced or underway in 10 of the 12 communities we track, with multiple mergers occurring in many cases. In our second round of site visits, we sought to explore how these arrangements were progressing and the implications of hospital mergers for local communities.

To many, hospital mergers were viewed as an important step toward restructuring local healthcare systems to become more efficient because they promised the rationalizing of excess capacity in local communities that contribute to high costs of care. However, to the residents of local communities, hospital mergers raised concerns about continued access to services and the potential loss of jobs and the redirection of charitable assets from their original purpose. Moreover, from a policy perspective, there were concerns that the efficiency gains from hospital mergers might be outweighed

---

The authors gratefully acknowledge the comments provided by Paul Ginsburg and Joy Grossman on earlier drafts of this chapter.

by gains in market power, which would allow hospitals to obtain higher prices for their services and withstand pressure to control costs.

Extensive literature on hospital mergers and their impact exists, but considerable debate over these effects continues. Some research suggests that hospital mergers produce efficiencies in local healthcare systems because they result in some reduced inpatient capacity and lowered utilization and they yield some cost savings (see for example, Bogue et al. 1995; Woolley 1989). Other research suggests, however, that hospital mergers result in higher prices because consolidation leaves hospitals in a stronger position to exert market power (Dranove and Ludwick 1999; Keeler, Melnick, and Zwanziger 1999; Simpson and Shin 1998). The latter suggestion is consistent with other studies that support the idea that under managed care, in particular, hospitals can negotiate higher prices if they have fewer competitors and greater market share (Melnick et al. 1992; Brooks, Dor, Wong 1997; Bamezai et al. 1999).

The CTS site visits contribute to our understanding of hospital mergers and their impact. Designed around a small but nationally representative sample of markets, the CTS allowed us to delve into specific cases of hospital mergers in local markets, while building a picture of hospital-merger activity across the United States. Moreover, the qualitative nature of the data allowed us to get behind the "end result" of the merger. In this way, we could explore the motivation for the strategy and the series of decisions about implementation that determine how hospital mergers take shape and how they affect communities.

We defined our sample to include all full-asset hospital mergers that had been announced or recently executed in our 12 communities or study sites during our first site visits from 1996 to 1997, which gave us a diverse sample of hospital mergers across a nationally representative set of markets. This resulted in a sample of 17 mergers in 10 communities (see Table 2.1 for a list of the mergers). The mergers varied in their stage of implementation: some already had been in progress, while others had just recently been announced. Three of the 17 mergers had come apart by our second site visits from 1998 to 1999.

Data on the mergers were collected through semistructured interviews, with protocols focusing on the objectives of the merger, the progress of implementation, and its impact. Special interview protocols were designed for the "failed mergers," focusing on what caused the merger to come apart and how hospitals proceeded to pursue the objectives of the merger afterward. Multiple respondents were interviewed for each case, including various respondents from the hospitals involved in the merger and respondents, who were selected to provide "vantage" perspectives, from other hospitals, health plans, and physician organizations in the market.

Responses were "triangulated" to validate the data and to allow all individual responses to be kept confidential. Secondary data, primarily from the American Hospital Association, were also employed to objectively measure the impact of the mergers on bed size, market share, and occupancy rates in our study sites.

In our analysis presented in this chapter, we describe hospitals' mergers and how they are implemented in the context of the market conditions at the time of our two site visits. We discuss the specific objectives sought through the merger and the successes and obstacles to implementation. In particular, we define the administrative and clinical functions that are merged and the extent to which mergers reduce capacity. We also describe the effect of mergers on hospitals' market power and competitive position in the local market. Finally, we draw on these findings to discuss the implications of hospital mergers for local communities in terms of their impact on the re-organization of care delivery and their expected effect on healthcare costs.

Findings

At the time of our 1996 to 1997 site visits, when these mergers had just been announced or begun implementation, hospitals confronted several significant pressures, most important of which was the growth—and anticipated continued growth—of managed care. Enrollment in HMOs and PPOs had grown significantly in many communities, increasing pressure for discounted payments and raising expectations about the proliferation of risk-contracting arrangements. The belief that both Medicare and Medicaid would dramatically increase reliance on managed care arrangements fueled these expectations, while recently announced direct cuts in Medicare reimbursement under the Balanced Budget Act of 1997 further threatened hospital revenues.

At the same time, national for-profit hospital chains—most prominently Columbia/HCA—were gaining force, and the threat of new entry loomed large in many communities (Kohn 2000). Similarly, national for-profit managed care companies were growing rapidly—in part because of the growth in managed care enrollment and in part because of acquisitions of their own—introducing new payers or boosting existing payers' bargaining power in the local market. In response to this competition, local health plans likewise pursued mergers and acquisitions that broadened their geographic scope in an effort to appeal to employers with an increasingly regional workforce (Grossman 2000). Together, these changes confronted local hospitals with new competitive threats in their traditional market areas and promised diminishing leverage in negotiations with payers.

This combination of pressures presented hospitals with a number of new challenges. In the most immediate sense, hospitals needed to find ways to protect their bottom line, by finding ways (1) to preserve revenue by staving off discounts and protecting their market share and (2) to control costs by streamlining operations. In the longer view, hospitals also sought to prepare for the coming of more extensive managed care, with increased reliance on risk contracting and more selective provider networks. To position themselves for these arrangements, hospitals sought to establish full-service provider networks that could build their leverage in contract negotiations and could coordinate clinical care and manage financial risk for the full spectrum of patient care. They also sought to secure key distinguishing services (e.g., neonatal intensive care services or the only Level 1 trauma service in the region) and/or significant geographic breadth, which would make them indispensable to local managed care networks (Kohn 2000).

Hospitals and Their Mergers

Hospitals viewed their mergers as a strategy to address many, if not all, of these goals. Despite all the attention to national for-profit hospital chains, especially at the time of our first site visits in 1996, most of the mergers in our study involved local not-for-profit hospitals merging with one another (see Table 2.1). The hospitals involved were among the largest and most prominent in their communities (e.g., Massachusetts General Hospital with 900+ beds, Brigham and Women's Hospital with 700+ beds in Boston, or the Cleveland Clinic Foundation Hospital with 900+ beds in Cleveland). In some cases, hospitals merged with one-time rivals (e.g., in Indianapolis, Methodist Health Group merged with Indiana University Medical Center to form Clarian Health Partners). In other cases, leading tertiary care institutions merged with smaller community hospitals (e.g., St. Barnabas Medical Center in Northern New Jersey or the Cleveland Clinic Foundation Hospital in Cleveland).

Although all of the cases in our study were full-asset mergers, hospitals took different approaches to these arrangements. Roughly half of the cases were structured as "mergers" or "acquisitions," where one hospital absorbed the assets and liabilities of the generally weaker institution. The other cases were structured as "consolidations," where both organizations were formally dissolved and together formed a new entity (Bogue et al. 1995). In these latter cases, the hospitals often kept their original names but joined together under the banner of a new system name (e.g., Partners HealthCare System, where Massachusetts General and Brigham and Women's Hospitals have maintained their own identities, or Clarian

Health Partners, where Methodist Health Group and Indiana University Medical Center have kept their own names.) This consolidation arrangement was common in mergers that involved two hospitals of similar size or reputation prior to the merger. This arrangement was also common among many academic medical centers in our study, apparently as a strategy to leverage the brand identity of the two institutions in the creation of a new system.

Despite these different structures, nearly every system in our study maintained some level of local hospital governance. In some cases, this involved local hospital representation on the parent company board. In most cases, it also involved maintaining local boards to serve an advisory or watchdog function. Absolute dissolution of local hospital governance was observed in only two cases, and both cases involved the acquisitions of for-profit hospitals that did not have community boards previously.

Merger Objectives

Hospital executives characterized their mergers to be motivated by two main objectives: (1) the desire to increase efficiency of their operations and (2) the desire to increase their market power relative to health plans and competitors. Objectives related to efficiency gains were noted with less frequency but were identified in all cases. These objectives focused on efforts to rationalize duplicative services and eliminate excess capacity to hold down operational costs. Efficiency gains were also expected through the efforts to "reengineer" the care delivery process across the partner hospitals in preparation for a managed-care-dominated system, which would reward managing the cost of care along the full continuum of services rather than simply reimbursing providers on a fee-for-service basis.

Objectives related to market power centered on efforts to consolidate market share and strengthen the hospitals' bargaining position relative to health plans. For example, many respondents described their mergers as a strategy to reduce competition in the local market, limiting the number of hospitals that they have to compete against for patient volume and for inclusion in health plans' provider networks. This was the strategy of the merger between one-time rivals; the hospitals contended that by combining forces, they would not only eliminate their most pressing competitive threat for market share, but they also would increase their indispensability in managed care contracts.

In many cases, respondents described the merger to be aimed at building a comprehensive service network and expanding the hospitals' geographic scope to attract greater volume and give them greater leverage with

Study Site	System	Hospitals Involved (bed size at time of merger)[1]	Year of Merger
Boston	Partners HealthCare System	Massachusetts General Hospital (899) Brigham and Women's Hospital (712)	1994
	The CareGroup	Beth Israel Hospital (447) New England Deaconess Hospital (314)	1996
	Boston Medical Center	Boston University Hospital (311) Boston City Hospital (282)	1995
Cleveland	Cleveland Clinic Health System	Cleveland Clinic Hospital (945) Meridia System (778) Fairview Health System (627)	1995
	University Hospital Health System	University Hospitals Health System (677) Bedford Community Hospital (110) Geauga Community Hospital (100)	1994
Greenville	Anderson Greenville Spartanburg System	Greenville Hospital System (1,203) Anderson Area Medical Center (445) Spartanburg Regional Medical Center (480)	Announced 1995, Failed 1996
Indianapolis	Clarian Health Partners	Methodist Health Group (924) Indiana University Medical Center (380) Riley Children's Hospital (230)	1997
Lansing	Sparrow Health System	Sparrow Health System (379) St. Lawrence Hospital (375)	1997
Little Rock	St. Vincent Health System	St. Vincent Health System (537) Columbia Doctors Hospital (308)	1998
Miami	Baptist Health System	Baptist Health System (392) South Miami Hospital (397) Homestead Hospital (120)	1995

1 AHA Annual Survey Database™ for Fiscal Year 1998, Health Forum, LLC, an American Hospital Association company, copyright 2000.

TABLE 2.1 *(continued)*

Study Site	System	Hospitals Involved (bed size at time of merger)[1]	Year of Merger
Miami	Baptist Health System[2]	Baptist Health System (909) Mercy Hospital (365)	Announced 1996, Failed 1998
	Tenet Healthcare	Tenet Healthcare (1,403 in Miami) North Shore Medical Center (320)	1997
Northern New Jersey	St. Barnabas Health Care System	St. Barnabas Medical Center (594) Newark Beth Israel Hospital (510) Irvington General Hospital (157) Union Hospital (201)	1995-1996
	Atlantic Health System	Morristown Memorial Hospital (637) Overlook Hospital (464) Mountainside Hospital (396)	1996
Orange County	St. Joseph's Health System	St. Joseph's Health System (728) Mission Hospital (202)	1994
	Tenet Healthcare	Tenet Healthcare (1,290 in Orange County) Fountain Valley Hospital (413) Garden Grove Hospital (167)	1996
Phoenix	Catholic HealthCare West	Catholic HealthCare West (493 in Phoenix) Samaritan Health System (1,348 in Phoenix)	Announced 1996, Failed 1997

2 Because the Baptist-Mercy merger was a subsequent merger that had a different outcome from the Baptist-South Miami and Homestead merger, it was considered as a distinct case in this study.

health plans. This strategy is evident in the merger of large tertiary care institutions with small community hospitals, in their effort to round out their service mix and to secure a steady referral base. In many cases, this strategy was also linked to an effort to expand urban hospitals' service areas into suburban areas in which they did not have a presence previously.

In some cases, mergers seemed to emerge from a reactive rather than a proactive strategy because hospitals feared being left at a disadvantage if they did not choose their partners early. In this respect, mergers gave rise to more mergers, which is a phenomenon observed in such markets as Boston, Cleveland, and northern New Jersey where multiple, distinct hospital mergers occurred in the course of a very short time period.

Merger Implementation

Operationalizing the merger strategy, and often-competing objectives, proved much more difficult than respondents anticipated. Tensions over control represented a significant obstacle to implementation and were the crux of the problem for the three failed mergers in our study. In two of these cases, the demise of the merger was linked to conflict over governance and leadership control. For example, in Miami, the merger of a Baptist and a Catholic hospital came apart because they disagreed over which partner's religious views, regarding reproductive health and end-of-life decisions, would dominate in the new system. In Phoenix, two long-standing rivals' attempt to merge fell through over discrepancies concerning the level of control that one partner was expected to relinquish in exchange for the assumption of its debt. In Greenville, three local hospitals planned to merge and form a new system, which would have captured an estimated 85 percent of inpatient admissions in the area. Although none of the hospitals involved was a public hospital, the question of the merger was put to area voters in a nonbinding ballot referendum. After a great deal of negative publicity sponsored largely by a competing local hospital, area residents expressed their opposition to the merger and, although the vote did not obligate them to do so, the hospitals walked away from the deal shortly thereafter.

Tensions over control and competing objectives have shaped the implementation of the mergers as well. The mergers we studied were fraught with conflict stemming from competing interests of the hospitals involved, culture clashes among the affiliated physicians, and conflicting demands from the community. These tensions were reflected in the decisions about what functions to consolidate and how to operationalize the merger.

Functions and Capacities Merged

Among the 14 hospitals in our study that proceeded with their mergers, extensive consolidation of administrative functions took place, but relatively little consolidation of clinical services or capacity occurred. In fact, although few closures and some downsizing occurred, many cases of

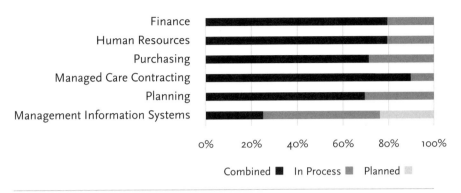

expansion of services and capacity took place as a result of the merger and the drive for greater market share and leverage.

Consolidation of Administrative Services. Many hospitals consolidated administrative functions shortly after the merger was implemented. As Figure 2.1 illustrates, most systems made quick progress combining functions such as finance, human resources, and purchasing, identifying these areas as the low-hanging fruit for quick efficiency gains. Many hospitals' prior experience with joint purchasing and/or outsourcing some of these administrative functions appears to have facilitated early consolidation in these areas.

Managed care contracting is another area that has seen significant progress, pointing toward the importance of managed-care–related goals in the merger strategy. Many hospitals moved rapidly to establish single signature contracts or some form of coordinated contracting across the hospitals in the system to leverage their new size with health plans. Although many hospitals continued to contract with health plans on an individual basis, they commonly centralized negotiation of these contracts across the merger partners in an effort to solidify their clout with health plans. In addition, many systems established coordinated contracting vehicles for the affiliated physicians across the system to bolster their clout in managed care contract negotiations. Some of these resulted in large entities, covering 3,000 to 3,500 physicians in their networks.

Notably, one key administrative function that was not as likely to have been merged was the hospitals' management information system (MIS). Although just under half of all of the cases reported that centralization of MIS was planned or already underway to some degree, this function had

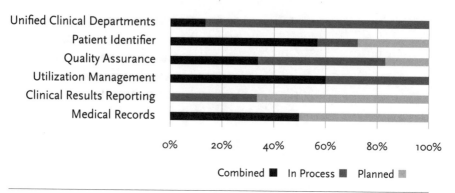

been combined in only two cases. MIS is probably the most challenging
administrative function to combine, given the investments that each hospital has made in its respective MIS and the likely differences between the
two systems. Moreover, in cases where the hospitals make the hard decision to merge their information systems, the implementation has been
difficult. For example, one system that merged its billing and reimbursement functions encountered problems, which left the system with an estimated $35 million in expired and uncollectable bills.

Consolidation of Clinical Functions. Overall, systems made less headway
with efforts to combine clinical services and clinical infrastructure, as illustrated in Figure 2.2. Although 10 of the 14 systems planned, and in
some cases had begun, to coordinate clinical services and support functions to some degree, most made only modest progress with these initiatives at the time of our second round of site visits. Some systems reported
that they have taken an explicitly decentralized approach to clinical services, noting that the geographic spread of the partners diminishes the value
of consolidation. Moreover, because one primary objective of many mergers is to build broad geographic networks, disincentives to consolidating
clinical services exist if it means abandoning services at some locations. In
addition, the inherent conflict this process creates among hospital partners, and physicians in particular, has led systems to approach this en-
deavor with caution. These initiatives also are the most visible to patients,
and most systems noted an interest in minimizing the impact of the
merger on the community.

Nevertheless, some systems had begun the process of clinical consolidation, generally starting with what functions are considered the least disruptive and those that are the most useful in managing care and risk-bearing contracts. As illustrated in Figure 2.2, one of the most commonly combined clinical function was patient identifiers; this function was combined in only four cases and was planned or in process in just three others. Respondents identified this area as one of the most immediately useful tools for managing care across the system. With a common identifier, the system can track episodes of care and develop outcomes data critical for managing risk contracts. Common medical records, however, were not observed in any of the cases at the time of our second round of site visits, although many systems noted that they would be interested in developing this function if and when viable automated records systems emerge.

In a handful of cases, utilization management and quality assurance have been combined, and this was planned or in process in a few other cases. These functions also feed into the care reengineering process and are essential to managed care relationships because they provide the means for systems to measure their performance and thereby control costs and negotiate with health plans. However, incompatibility of information systems pose limits to these endeavors and slowed consolidation of these functions. Some systems took steps toward this goal by sharing information across hospitals, but they had not begun to formally combine quality assurance and utilization management.

The most advanced and difficult aspect of clinical consolidation moves beyond centralization of the infrastructure to manage care delivery to the consolidation of clinical services. Only one system in our study had fully unified clinical departments under single department chiefs. More than half of the remaining systems reported partial consolidation of clinical services, with the appointment of systemwide chairs for only selected departments or the establishment of other forms of more loosely structured arrangements. Services most readily combined centered on support services and hospital-based physicians, such as radiology and pathology. Two systems also reported consolidation of their behavioral health programs and two others consolidated pediatrics. Other systems reported some degree of centralization in neurology, orthopedics, obstetrics, and neonatology. Even in cases where only partial consolidation of clinical services had occurred, hospitals experienced substantial disruption and physician defection. For example, in the merger of Sparrow and St. Lawrence hospitals in Lansing, the consolidation of the obstetrics departments caused unrest among physicians, and many obstetricians left to affiliate with the competing system in the market. The most dramatic case in our study was observed in the consolidation of Beth Israel and Deaconess Medical Center. The hospitals appointed single department heads and consolidated services rapidly, leading to physician defections and, consequently, steep financial losses. Deaconess's anesthesiologists resigned en masse after the departments were united, and several prominent surgeons who worked with them—including a famed liver transplant team—announced that they would move to a rival hospital.

In contrast, the one system that pursued fully unified clinical departments, Boston Medical Center, met with greater success. Both hospitals were in severe financial distress at the time of their merger and set clear goals for combining clinical staffs from the outset. Moreover, the fact that the hospitals had largely complementary services meant that this could be accomplished with less conflict than elsewhere.

In fact, although hospitals with greater geographic overlap may seem to be able to make more progress with clinical consolidation, this does not play out in our study. For example, Clarian Health Partners is a merger of two hospitals in close geographic proximity, but difficulties with combining the physician cultures of an academic medical center and a large community hospital stymied efforts to combine clinical functions. Rather, the systems that did the most to combine clinical functions seem to be those that had largely complementary service areas, where little conflict of interest exists.

Similarly, contrary to what might be expected, a direct correlation between the amount of time elapsed and the degree of clinical consolidation does not appear to exist. Some systems that have been in place for three to four years had some of the least clinical consolidation, while other newer mergers made more progress in this regard. Nevertheless, many of the systems viewed more extensive clinical consolidation to be on the horizon and expected that given the difficulty involved, these efforts will take more time. One large system reported that it expects it will take three to five years to accomplish its clinical consolidation goals. Other systems explicitly stayed away from establishing timelines, although they acknowledged plans for clinical consolidation.

Consolidation of Capacity. In part because of the limited clinical consolidation and in part because of efforts to minimize the visibility and direct impact of the mergers on the local community, limited reduction of capacity has been reported in the mergers we studied. Overall, expansion of capacity appears as much as reduction of capacity as a result of hospital mergers.

We observed downsizing and closures in 8 of the 14 cases of mergers in our study. We noted only three cases of closures, and all of them had been planned from the outset and involved obsolete facilities that would have required substantial investments to upgrade. Downsizing occurred in five cases, with reductions of approximately 10 to 20 percent of the pre-merger bed size, although it is unclear that these changes can be directly associated with the merger itself since many hospitals were actively eliminating beds during this period.

At the same time, expansions in 6 of the 14 cases occurred, mostly in terms of outpatient capacity, but some inpatient capacity expansion was observed as well. Some of the greatest expansion occurred in Cleveland, where the two newly consolidated systems have been adding high-end specialty services at outlying community hospitals in a race to establish loyalty and referral relationships. Again, it is unclear that these expansions can be directly related to the merger itself since this was a common competitive strategy at the time. For example, in Greenville, where an attempted merger failed, the three hospitals involved in the proposed deal have made similar expansions in key services such as cardiology, radiation/oncology, and other ambulatory services targeted as revenue enhancing. Nevertheless, expansions, such as those observed in Cleveland and other markets, appear to have been facilitated by the relationships established under their mergers.

Effects of Mergers on Hospitals' Market Power

Although hospital mergers appear to have produced limited clinical consolidation or reduction of capacity, it is undeniable that mergers have had an impact on local markets as a result of increased concentration of ownership. Figure 2.3 illustrates how the concentration of market share (as measured by total adjusted hospital admissions) has changed in the 12 study sites over the past few years. Mergers produced increasingly concentrated market share in several sites, with the biggest changes taking place in Cleveland and Lansing. Between 1994 and 1997, Cleveland jumped from being an unconcentrated market to almost becoming considered highly concentrated, with the multiple mergers involving the Cleveland Clinic and University Hospitals Health System. Subsequent acquisitions by these two systems, indeed, have pushed the market into the highly concentrated category.

The Lansing hospital market, which was already highly concentrated in 1994 with just three hospitals serving the community, became even more highly concentrated in 1996 as a result of the merger of two of its hospitals. Interestingly, however, little concern was voiced locally or at the federal level about this increase in consolidation, apparently in part because the

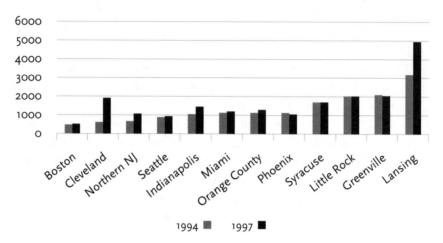

Note: Concentration is measured by a Herfindahl Index based on total adjusted hospital admissions. A market with a Herfindahl Index of less than 1000 is considered unconcentrated, those between 1000 and 1800 are considered moderately concentrated, and those over 1800 are considered highly concentrated (U.S. Department of Justice and the Federal Trade Commission. "Horizontal Merger Guidelines." Issued: April 2, 1992; Revised: April 8, 1997. Section 1.5)

merger involved the acquisition of a financially weak hospital by a stronger local entity and in part because the services and geographic areas of the partners were largely complementary.

Based on our study, it appears that mergers have been successful at helping hospitals solidify, and in some cases improve, their position in the market. Generally, respondents indicated that mergers have helped long-standing dominant hospitals to stave off declines in volume and, in some cases, attain modest increases. Sometimes, this increased volume came at the expense of their merger partners, resulting in greater concentration of volume at the leading hospital or hospitals in the system. In other cases, the system was reportedly able to expand volume across the affiliated hospitals as a result of the merger strategy. A net gain in volume for the system as a whole was noted in markets, such as Cleveland and Northern New Jersey, where smaller community hospitals reportedly were able to attract greater patient volume and build market share as a result of the merger. Some attributed these gains to the availability of new services at the community hospitals that were facilitated through the merger; others identified the new "branding" of the community hospital with the name of the highly regarded tertiary care institution as an important contributor to the increase in volume.

A similar dynamic led the hospitals involved in mergers to successfully expand their geographic scope. For example, two Boston-based systems, Partners HealthCare System and The CareGroup, expanded their service areas into eastern Massachusetts and New Hampshire because the new relationship between hospitals in outlying areas and prestigious tertiary-care institutions helped the community hospitals to attract patients from a broader geographic area. Respondents noted a similar experience in Cleveland, where local hospitals have expanded their service areas into eastern Ohio and western Pennsylvania as a result of recent mergers. Hospitals in Indianapolis, Little Rock, and Northern New Jersey also appear to have successfully expanded their reach in other parts of the state in this way. These expansions have been important to help maintain volume and to achieve greater leverage in contract negotiations with managed care plans. Interestingly, the hospitals involved in the failed mergers in our study also achieved some expansion of their geographic reach during this period, although generally this occurred as a result of new affiliations or mergers that they entered into subsequently.

Overall, respondents report that mergers have helped hospitals improve their leverage with managed care plans, which was one of the key objectives of the merger strategy. The majority of the systems we studied appear to have strengthened their bargaining position as a result of the merger. Many noted that the systems were now clearly "must-have" providers in managed care contracts and the merger allowed them to secure new contracts and better contract terms in many instances. For example, shortly after the merger was complete, Cleveland Clinic Health System was able to secure a new multiyear, single signature contract with Aetna, which had better rates and contract terms than the associated hospitals had previously. Similarly, respondents from other markets noted that hospitals are in a stronger position in managed care contract negotiations because of their unified front.

However, not all of the systems secured the clout they hoped for through their mergers. For example, in both Cleveland and Little Rock, hospitals that had previously been excluded from key contracts remained locked-out of these arrangements, despite their improved market position under the merger. In addition, hospitals have found that although the merger has helped increase their leverage for contracting as a system, this has not typically translated into increases in reimbursement. Rather, the gain in market power is seen in the fact that mergers have reportedly helped hospitals stave off further discounts and prevent the erosion of market power they have been experiencing over the past several years. Notably, however, these successes occurred at a time when vigorous consumer backlash also existed against managed care, which boosted providers' leverage to push back on pricing (see Chapter 1). Moreover, note that in some cases hospitals' increased leverage appears to have been held in check by countervailing forces that have prevented them from exerting excessive power in the market. Lansing is perhaps the best example of this phenomenon. Although the hospital market is now concentrated in just two local systems, their power is held in check by the countervailing force of a highly concentrated payer market—70 percent of which is held by a single health plan—and a highly concentrated employer market that has been very aggressive in its demands to control costs. This creates a competitive dynamic that limits the ability of the hospital systems to exercise their market power and drive up prices. The same might be said about Boston, where the healthcare system could be described as a bilateral monopoly with concentrated power of both health plans and provider systems holding one another in check. In the absence of their mergers, however, it is clear that these hospitals would have been in a much weaker position to negotiate contract terms given the degree of consolidation that has emerged among plans in these markets and in the majority of our study sites (Grossman 2000).

For some hospitals, the gains in market leverage were offset to some degree by the costs of implementing the merger strategy. In many cases, the merger involved a financially strong hospital assuming the debt of financially weaker institutions, which put a strain on the system. Hospitals found that their mergers also exacted a cost in terms of distracting management from the external environment, as they needed to attend to internal implementation issues. In addition, we were told in many cases that the merger was much more costly than expected. Although some up-front investments were anticipated, systems found that it was taking much more time and money to establish the infrastructure to support the new system. Partners HealthCare System, for example, had estimated savings of $240 million from the merger and reported savings of $160 million within three years of implementing the merger; however, new overhead costs associated with infrastructure for the system are now estimated at $50 million to $60 million annually, which are offsetting these gains.

Conclusion

Our study suggests that, at least in the near term, while mergers have yielded important benefits for the hospitals involved, they have translated neither into the hoped-for efficiency gains nor the feared excessive market power. Efficiency gains have been limited by a number of factors. First, hospitals have been reluctant to make significant changes in the organization of their care delivery system that will have visible effects on affiliated physicians or the community. As a result, although hospitals have made strides with integrating "back-room" functions such as purchasing and finance, few have taken steps to consolidate clinical services and capacity, which would yield more significant efficiency gains.

Second, hospitals' reluctance to make dramatic changes in the organization of care was reinforced during this period by managed care's failure to develop as anticipated. At the time that the hospitals in our study first pursued their mergers, the expectations were that healthcare markets were moving toward more tightly managed insurance products, which relied on selective provider networks and risk-based payment arrangements to manage the cost of care. Hospitals sought to prepare for this changing environment by establishing linkages with multiple hospitals and physicians that would allow them to manage the full spectrum of patient services in order to accept financial risk for patient care and to increase their leverage in contracting with health plans. However, as hospitals began to assemble the pieces for this strategy, consumer backlash against managed care halted the expected march toward selective networks and risk-based payment (see Chapter 1). As a result, hospitals confronted diminishing pressure to "re-engineer" the care delivery system in their communities.

In an environment where broad provider networks and ease of consumer access became so highly valued, hospitals indeed encountered added disincentives to clinical or capacity consolidation. In the absence of significant levers to manage the cost of care, health plans continued to push for provider discounts while pursuing a strategy of geographic expansion and consolidation. To maintain leverage with plans, hospitals sought to match health plans' broadening geographic reach and faced disincentives to reorganize services or reduce capacity in a manner that would diminish their geographic presence. At the same time, this response to health plan behavior fueled a competitive dynamic among hospitals, whereby hospitals increasingly compete on the outskirts of their traditional service areas to attract greater volume and expand market share. This dynamic added to the disincentives to rationalize services across the merger partners when they contributed to the system's geographic breadth. In fact, in many instances, mergers have been important vehicles for hospitals to expand services rather than reduce them.

While efficiency gains have been limited, mergers have helped hospitals to increase their market power. With newly consolidated leverage, hospitals involved in mergers achieved a stronger negotiating position with health plans and, in many cases, were able to stave off further declines in reimbursement. It is important to note, however, that although mergers have helped hospitals stem the erosion of their reimbursement rates, they have not yielded the power to dictate prices or contract terms, which would indicate excessive leverage. Rather, it appears that hospitals' increased market power has been held in check by the countervailing force of concentrated power on the part of health plans. In this respect, mergers allowed hospitals to balance the greater concentration among health plans but did not put them in a position to unilaterally control the market.

Nevertheless, it is important to recognize that hospitals' increased leverage—both as a result of their mergers and increasingly favorable market conditions—has put them in a stronger position to withstand pressure to achieve efficiencies. From the perspective of the local community, this outcome may be viewed as positive because it has helped to prevent the dramatic reorganization of the delivery system, preserving local access to services and protecting local jobs and charitable assets. However, from a broader societal perspective, these benefits come at the expense of the opportunity to achieve more significant reductions in healthcare costs.

What remains to be seen is how the effects of mergers play out over time, particularly as the economy worsens. Hospitals likely will face renewed pressure to control costs, which may prompt them to more aggressively pursue the efficiencies planned under their merger strategy. Given the concentration of ownership that has emerged in many markets and the time elapsed since the mergers were first established, hospitals may be poised to make much more rapid changes in the delivery system than previously. On the other hand, the increased market power that hospitals achieved through their mergers may have produced sufficient leverage to withstand significant levels of pressure for such change and may indeed push the system toward other solutions to control the cost of care.

CHAPTER 3

Blue Plans: Playing the Blues No More

Joy M. Grossman, Ph.D., and Bradley C. Strunk

Introduction

The "Blues" are not just any health plan. Taken together, local member companies of the Blue Cross and Blue Shield Association (BCBSA) have insured millions of Americans for nearly three quarters of a century. Throughout their history, they have been witness to and played a role in countless changes in the healthcare system. Today, 46 Plans provide healthcare coverage to 79 million people or one in four Americans, making them the largest private payer in the U.S. (BCBSA 2001). Their collective enrollment in government insurance programs and their share of Medicare claims processing far surpasses any other plan (BCBSA 2001). Their combined enrollment in HMO products makes them the largest provider of such products in the United States (InterStudy 2000). As Rosemary Stevens wrote in her foreword to *The Blues: A History of the Blue Cross and Blue Shield System* (Cunningham and Cunningham 1997): "One cannot understand the peculiar, constantly evolving, even Byzantine challenges of health care organization and financing in the United States in the twentieth century without also understanding the role, the changes, and the

The authors are grateful to Harry Cain, Nancy Chockley, and Roger Taylor for valuable insights into the evolution of the Blues. The authors would like to thank the following individuals as well: Robert Hurley, William Winkenwerder, Cara Lesser, Paul Ginsburg, Lawrence Brown, and Jon Christianson for helpful comments on earlier drafts of this chapter.

continuing dilemmas of the Blue Cross and Blue Shield Plans, past and present."

These Plans have played a unique and central role in local communities. Amid an environment of rapidly rising costs and little insurance coverage, the Blues entered an arena where commercial insurance companies had been reluctant to go, establishing themselves as the first prepaid health insurance plans over 70 years ago. Each individual Plan developed locally and independently, with local representation on its board of directors. A defining characteristic of these early Plans and their leaders was their commitment to community service and the provision of public benefit. As a consequence, the Plans operated on a not-for-profit basis, accepted all persons who desired insurance coverage, and used community rating to set uniform premiums without regard for individual enrollee health status or risk factors. Local accountability and community mission were indeed a hallmark of the early Plans.

The early Blues also enjoyed advantages from a number of other defining characteristics. In return for the public benefit they provided, they were subject to special regulatory treatment, which provided tax benefits and other advantages. Also, they had close ties to providers, rooted in their origins as provider-sponsored organizations, which yielded broad networks and provider discounts. Finally, each Plan benefited from the exclusive use of the Blue Cross and Blue Shield trademarks in their designated service area, eliminating competition from other Blue Plans. The Blues were able to leverage their early presence along with these unique conditions to develop the value of their brand name and to gain and maintain a dominant position in local markets (Frech 1996).

Despite the dominance they achieved, the Blues have never been immune to the pressures of a changing operating environment. While they have struggled with and responded successfully to pressures from regulators, purchasers, and competitors over their long history, the process of change and adaptation has made them less distinct from their competitors over time (Cunningham and Cunningham 1997; Brown 1997). In particular, adaptation has led to a diminishing of their community mission and public-benefit role. For example, in the 1950s, under competitive pressure from commercial insurers, many Plans abandoned community rating—a hallmark of their community focus—and switched to experience rating when setting premiums for group business.

The developments in healthcare organization and financing of the past 15-20 years have posed new challenges for the Blues and have diminished their dominance in many markets. There has been rapid growth in employers' dependence on managed care and the rise of national for-profit managed care companies, increasing reliance on self-insurance among employers, and greater demand by national employers for multistate accounts. At times, the Blues have been slow to respond to these pressures or have made serious missteps, with many Plans losing significant local market share (Cunningham and Cunningham 1997). For example, during the late 1980s and early 1990s, some Plans suffered serious financial problems and several high-profile management mishaps occurred (U.S. GAO 1994). Critics continue to question the Blues' ability to compete effectively in a managed care environment despite the benefits of still substantial market share, a strong brand name, and longstanding relationships with providers (Friedman 1998).

While much has been written about the Blues throughout this period, few systematic studies about them in the era of managed care exist (Cunningham and Cunningham 1997; Friedman 1998; Cain Brothers 1997). This chapter presents our analysis, which seeks to fill this gap in the literature. It uses data from HSC's 1998-1999 CTS site visits to explore how the Blues are positioned to compete in today's healthcare market and their strategic responses to current pressures. Given the importance of their role in the market, we also examine the implications of their market position and strategies for consumers and policymakers. In particular, we consider the extent to which the current strategies of the Blues could lead to erosion of the benefits they provide to consumers at the local level, and whether or not policymakers should be concerned.

This chapter describes the study design and the 14 Blue Cross and Blue Shield Plans included in the study sample; reports on the market pressures facing Blue Plans as they compete in today's market; explores the ways in which the Blues continue to be uniquely positioned in the market relative to their competitors—large market share, broad networks and product array, longevity in local markets, membership in the BCBSA, and regulatory treatment; and assesses how these characteristics affect their relationships with providers and purchasers. In addition, it discusses the strategies being pursued by the Blues. Two strategic responses to market pressures have potential implications for consumers: (1) decisions about whether to cover hard-to-insure populations and (2) mergers and related for-profit conversions. It concludes with a discussion of the potential costs and benefits of the Blues' strategies for consumers in local communities and implications for public policy.

Study Design

This chapter is based on interviews completed during the second round of CTS site visits to 12 communities or study sites, which were conducted between June 1998 and February 1999.

Sample of Blue Plans

This analysis focuses on all 14 of the Blue Cross and Blue Shield Plans operating in the 12 CTS study sites (see Table 3.1 for a complete listing). In two sites, Orange County and Seattle, the Blue Cross Plan and the Blue Shield Plan remain separate organizations and actively compete against each other.

A strength of this study is that the sample of nationally representative health insurance markets allows for a systematic examination of Blue Plans located across the country. The 14 Plans represent a quarter of the 53 Plans that were members of the BCBSA at the end of 1998. The study Plans are in states that are equally divided among the four Census regions: Northeast, South, Midwest, and West. At the time of the site visits, there were 13 Plans that acted on a not-for-profit basis, eight of which were organized as non-profit entities under special enabling statutes and the other five as mutual companies. (Throughout the rest of this chapter, the term "not-for-profit" will be used to refer to both nonprofit and mutual companies) . One Plan, Blue Cross of California, operated as a for-profit company and was owned by the publicly traded WellPoint Health Networks, Inc. Three Plans had wholly owned for-profit HMO subsidiaries. Six of the 14 Plans were subsidiaries of parent companies that also operate subsidiaries in other service areas. The most well known of these parent companies are Anthem, Inc., which is the parent to two plans in this sample (Anthem BCBS of Indiana and Anthem BCBS of Ohio) and the aforementioned WellPoint. The Plans are also differentiated by number of enrollees, which ranged from around 670,000 in Blue Cross and Blue Shield of Central New York to 4.7 million in Blue Cross of California at the time of the site visits.

Data Collection

Information on the 14 Plans was gathered through interviews with 33 Blue Plan respondents. In eight of the 12 study sites, a minimum of three Blue Plan respondents were interviewed in each site; in the remaining four sites, either one or two respondents were interviewed. Respondents usually included a senior executive such as the CEO; a marketing executive; and, when possible, a medical director and/or network executive. In each market, other key players were interviewed to provide triangulation on the responses of Blue Plan respondents. A total of 95 "vantage" interviews were conducted, with an average of eight interviews per site. Vantage respondents included competing plans, hospitals, physician organizations, employers, and in five sites, state insurance regulators. Several interviews with

Study Site	Blue Cross and Blue Shield Plan	Corporate Parent	Profit Status of Parent	Service Area of Corporate Parent*
Boston	Blue Cross and Blue Shield of Massachusetts		Nonprofit	State
Cleveland	Anthem Blue Cross and Blue Shield of Ohio	Anthem, Inc.	Mutual	Multiple regions
Greenville	Blue Cross and Blue Shield of South Carolina		Mutual	State
Indianapolis	Anthem Blue Cross and Blue Shield of Indiana	Anthem, Inc.	Mutual	Multiple regions
Lansing	Blue Cross and Blue Shield of Michigan		Nonprofit	State
Little Rock	Arkansas Blue Cross Blue Shield		Mutual (For-profit HMO subsidiary)	State
Miami	Blue Cross and Blue Shield of Florida		Mutual	State
Northern New Jersey	Horizon Blue Cross and Blue Shield of New Jersey		Nonprofit (For-profit HMO subsidiary)	State
Orange County	Blue Cross of California	WellPoint Health Networks, Inc.	Publicly offered for-profit	Multiple regions
Phoenix	Blue Shield of California		Nonprofit	State
	Blue Cross and Blue Shield of Arizona		Nonprofit	State
Seattle	Premera Blue Cross	Premera Blue Cross	Nonprofit	Single region
	Regence Blue Shield	The Regence Group	Nonprofit	Single region
Syracuse	Blue Cross and Blue Shield of Central New York	Excellus, Inc.	Nonprofit (For-profit HMO subsidiary)	Within state

* Represents the corporate parent's service area for health insurance products sold under the BCBS trademark.

recognized experts also were done, including individuals affiliated with the BCBSA who provided a national perspective on Blue Plans.

To assess the role of Blue Plans in local markets, respondents were asked to comment on:

1. the current market position of the Blue Plan(s);
2. the pressures that were driving change among the Plans;
3. the advantages and disadvantages the Plans had in responding to these pressures; and
4. the competitive strategies being pursued by the Plans.

Although all of the Plans had service areas that were larger than the local CTS study site, respondents were asked to frame their answers in the context of the local market.

Several additional sources of data helped in this study. Findings from the first and second rounds of the CTS site visits provide an understanding of the competitive environments in each of the 12 study sites (Grossman 2000; Kohn 2000; Lesser and Ginsburg 2000; Kohn et al. 1997; Center for Studying Health System Change 1999). Background information on the Plans, such as corporate structure and product characteristics, was obtained from each Plan directly and/or through secondary sources. Baseline information was also available from the first round of interviews with the study plans. To allow for additional triangulation on the findings, trade publications were monitored throughout the study period for news about Blue Plans across the country.

Pressures Facing the Blues

The Blues' competitive strategies—including decisions about which products to offer, provider contracting strategies, and whether to merge with other plans—are affected by a number of important market and firm-specific factors (Grossman 2000). Market factors include purchaser demands, regulatory pressures, and the structure of the local health insurance market. Factors internal to Blue Plans include BCBSA rules, organizational culture, financial position, and access to capital. This section explores the most acute pressures facing the Blues in today's market.

General Market Pressures Facing Health Plans

In today's healthcare market, health plans, including the Blues, are facing a number of significant external pressures (Grossman 2000; Lesser and Ginsburg 2000). Over the past five years or so, there has been increasing purchaser demand for broad networks and less-restrictive managed care products, part of a broader documented managed care backlash, as well as more demand by multisite employers for broad geographic coverage. Greater competition has also surfaced from other health plans—particularly national managed care companies—that threaten to enter markets and take away market share from the Blues and other local plans. Finally, more recently, because underlying health care costs were increasing more rapidly than premiums over the past several years, all health plans have been feeling a squeeze on margins, and the Blues are no exception. This has meant more disciplined pricing and more targeted entry and exit of business lines than during the prior several years, when plans were focused on expanding market share rather than protecting margins. Blue Plan respondents confirmed that these pressures were affecting the Blues' strategic decision making at the time of the study.

Changes in the Regulation of the Blues and BCBSA Operating Rules

Traditionally, the Blues enjoyed favorable regulatory treatment in return for providing public benefit, although the degree of both regulation and public benefit varied significantly by state. To some extent, this variation was related to whether Plans were structured as nonprofits under special enabling statutes or as mutual companies, which tend to be regulated more like commercial insurance companies and have fewer benefits or obligations. All Blue Plans benefited from special federal and state tax treatment, and some received mandated provider discounts in states with hospital-rate regulation. In return, the Blue Plans frequently served as "insurer-of-last-resort" (i.e., covering all applicants regardless of health status) or sometimes applied community rating to the full population (i.e., basing premiums on the average expected costs of the entire risk pool). Other related regulations existed to ensure access and affordability, such as requirements for open enrollment, premium regulation for some or all products, and restrictions on the level of plan reserves.

The regulatory playing field, however, has been evolving toward a more level one for quite some time. In 1986, the Blues lost the right to a full exemption from federal income taxes; however, they can still receive a partial deduction under certain conditions (Forgione 1999). In addition, a number of Blue Plan respondents indicated that the insurer-of-last-resort requirements for their Plan—a fundamental way in which many of the Blues fulfilled their community service—were removed in the 1980s or earlier. As of 1991, only four study Plans were still subject to differential regulation in the individual and/or small group markets (U.S. GAO 1994). These regulations included open enrollment and partial or pure community rating. All of these Plans, with the exception of BCBS of Michigan, noted that the requirements specific to the Blues were replaced by state individual and small-group market insurance reforms in the early 1990s, which required all health plans to participate in ensuring access to coverage.

Some fundamental changes at the BCBSA have also occurred, which dramatically affect the way the Blues operate. In 1991, the BCBSA tightened its financial oversight of member Plans and revised its minimum surplus requirements, partially in response to the insolvency of the West Virginia Blue Plan (U.S. GAO 1994). Then, in 1994, the BCBSA took the unprecedented step of allowing investor ownership of Blue Plans, ending its longstanding requirement that each plan must act on a not-for-profit basis (Cunningham and Cunningham 1997). Prior to 1994, the BCBSA had stipulated that the corporate parents of member Plans operate on a not-for-profit basis, whether structured as a nonprofit or a mutual company (U.S. GAO 1994). For-profit subsidiaries, however, were allowed.

What It Means To Be "Blue" Today

Data from this study indicate that Blue Plans in the United States are well positioned, in terms of market share and product mix, to confront the pressures of today's market and a changing operating environment. These and other characteristics that have traditionally differentiated the Blues from their competitors continue to benefit them today, although certain characteristics, in some respects, are also weaknesses that continue to challenge each Plan.

Characteristics of the Blues

Large market share. Most Plans continue to maintain a strong position in local markets. Looking across all products, market respondents consider the Blues to be the dominant health plan with the largest market share in seven of our 12 study sites (see Table 3.2). Of these seven Plans, those that operate in Lansing, Little Rock, Syracuse, and Greenville stand out as having almost complete dominance in their markets with few competitors close in size; the first two Plans each have market shares of at least 50 percent in the states they cover. The Plans in Indianapolis, Northern New Jersey, and Seattle have the largest overall share in their markets, but they face more substantial competition from other health plans.

In the remaining five sites, the Blues are not the largest health plan but are still major competitors with significant market share. In most cases, in these sites, a number of health plans, including the Blues, have near-equal market share and jockey for the top slot. Only two study Plans are

Overall Market Position of Blue Plans	Local versus National Competitors	Overall Market Concentration (all health insurance products)	HMO Penetration*	Blues' HMO Market Position
Markets where the Blues are dominant in terms of overall market position				
Greenville	Mixed	Concentrated	Low	Leader
Indianapolis	Local	Concentrated	Low	Distant competitor
Lansing	Local	Concentrated	High	Close competitor
Little Rock	Mixed	Concentrated	Low	Leader
Northern New Jersey	National	Fragmented	Low	Close competitor
Seattle	Local	Concentrated	Low	Close competitor
Syracuse	Local	Concentrated	Low	Close competitor
Markets where the Blues are major competitors in terms of overall market position				
Boston	Local	Concentrated	High	Close competitor
Cleveland	Mixed	Concentrated	Low	Distant competitor
Miami	National	Fragmented	High	Close competitor
Orange County	National	Fragmented	High	Distant competitor
Phoenix	National	Fragmented	High	Distant competitor

Note: Blues' overall market position, HMO market position, and local versus national competitors based on CTS site visit interviews. Overall concentration determined using CTS Health Insurance Followback Survey and site visit data. HMO penetration based on estimates as of January 1, 1999 from The InterStudy County Surveyor.

* Above or below the mean for U.S. metropolitan areas with populations over 200,000.

significantly smaller than the other major competitors in the market. Blue Shield of California lags behind other plans in Orange County, including Blue Cross of California. Anthem BCBS of Ohio is unique because only in 1997 did it acquire the license to cover Cleveland as a Blue Plan. The BCBSA took the license away from the plan that still dominates that market—Medical Mutual of Ohio.

While the Blues typically offer a wide range of products, their strong overall market position in all sites can be attributed to their dominance in the PPO and indemnity product markets. They are much less likely to be the leading provider of HMO products. This means that the Blues are more likely to be dominant in those sites with lower-than-average HMO penetration than in those sites with higher-than-average HMO penetration.

Broad networks, wide product array, and longevity in the market. In almost every site, respondents indicated that the Blues have the broadest networks among all competing health plans. These broad networks serve as platforms that allow the Blues to offer a broad range of products including indemnity, PPO, HMO, and POS products. Respondents viewed this in contrast to many managed care companies that specialize in a single product line and then fill out their product array to satisfy large purchasers. Also, in all markets studied, the Blues have typically been in operation much longer than most other health plans. Therefore, the history of each local market is inextricably intertwined with the history of the Blue Plan or Plans that currently operate there.

BCBSA membership. Members are independent plans that are affiliated through the BCBSA. BCBSA provides services to those member Plans but does not act as a corporate parent; Plan interests are represented on the BCBSA board of directors and decisions are made by member vote. The association itself does not sell insurance. Through licensing agreements administered by the BCBSA, each Plan enjoys the right to use the Blue Cross and Blue Shield brand names and trademarks to distinguish themselves from their competitors. The licensing agreements offer each Plan an exclusive service area to sell branded products, ruling out competition among Blue Plans for branded products. BCBSA provides a number of services that help coordinate member Plans' coverage of enrollees across the country. For example, it administers the Federal Employees Health Benefits Program and the popular Blue Card program, which provides traveling enrollees with access to a nationwide network, and it helps service multistate employers who want a single contract across geographic areas (U.S. GAO 1994).

Minor regulatory differences. Because of the changes in the regulatory environment facing the Blues, respondents in this study perceived that differential regulation is no longer a distinguishing characteristic of most Blue Plans. Some Plans reported that they continue to be subject to differential regulation, including favorable tax treatment and regulatory burdens such as rate review, but most did not view these regulations as having a substantial impact, either positive or negative, on their ability to compete. Generally, regulations that are unique to the Blues are much less extensive today than the kind of regulation they have faced in the past. Often, Plans are subject to them because they are nonprofits, mutual companies, or are domiciled in state, rather than because they are Blue.

In the 12 study sites, only one Plan, BCBS of Michigan, is still being regulated as a "quasi-public utility." It is the only Plan in the study that is still required to be the insurer-of-last-resort. The state of Michigan also remains quite active in regulating many other aspects of its operations, including control of the membership of the Plan's board of directors: State law specifies all the interests that must be represented and who has a say in selecting the members.

The Advantages and Disadvantages of Being "Blue"

Relationships with providers. Respondents in all but two sites noted that the Blues' large market share gives them considerable market clout with providers. Even the Blues that are not dominant have significant leverage in setting payment rates. Perhaps the phrase used most often by respondents to describe the Blues was the "800-pound gorilla" in the market. Most providers—hospitals and physicians—participate in the Blues networks, and many get significant volume from Blues contracts. One national observer pointed out that the Blues benefit from contracts that give them discounts across all of their products. Historically, many Blue Plans had explicit "most-favored-nation" clauses in their provider contracts, which guaranteed them the lowest payment rates in the market. At least four study Plans still have such clauses, but the terms may be enforced only periodically. For example, BCBS of Central New York exercised the clause when a local HMO negotiated lower rates with physicians. Similarly, BCBS of South Carolina exercised the clause when a national for-profit HMO got lower rates.

Respondents did not report uniformly that all Blue Plans pay the lowest price in the market. Respondents in some markets indicated that, despite their clout, the Blues appear willing to pay more than other health plans that are demanding what providers perceive to be unreasonably low rates. Alternatively, Blue Plans may find that responding regularly to situations where lower rates are offered to other plans is not worth the effort, particularly if those plans have small market share and are not perceived as a threat, as suggested with the only periodic enforcement of the most-favored-nation clauses.

Suggestions were made that the Blues' relative advantages with providers are eroding. A few respondents at competing health plans, as well as national observers, noted that other managed care plans are increasingly successful at cutting into the leverage the Blues have over providers. In Northern New Jersey, for example, the increase in Aetna U.S. Healthcare's market share as a result of mergers with Prudential and NYLCare is seen as giving that plan the type of clout with providers that Horizon BCBS of New Jersey has enjoyed.

One downside of large market share, particularly in combination with broad networks, is that it makes the Blues a visible target for those unhappy with them, including providers. Given the large number of providers in the Blues' networks, they are more likely to resist or publicly complain about the Blues' efforts to impose rate cuts, even in markets where relationships with providers are relatively friendly. Across a number of markets, when periodic adjustments in the physician fee schedule result in rate cuts, they are regularly met with well-publicized outcry. However, because of the importance of the Blues products, physicians generally do not leave the network, although in some of the 12 study sites, stories have been circulating more recently about hospitals and physician groups threatening to terminate contracts with the Blues as well as with other plans. On some occasions, the Blues are responsive to provider concerns. For example, in Little Rock, complaints from doctors several years ago about the inadequacy of clinical data and payment delays caused Arkansas BCBS to quickly abandon a new payment initiative based on quality measures.

National observers noted that providers are also more likely to resist attempts by the Blues to pursue managed care initiatives that result in restricted networks of providers—for example, those that feature low-cost or high-quality providers. Unlike new entrants that can form narrow managed care networks from the start, the Blues have to *deselect* providers in order to create such networks. As in the case of the Blues' market share, this raises the potential for provider resistance and a general souring of relationships. Even trimming the network at the margin can elicit bad press, as was the case with one Blue Plan that canceled contracts with a small number of physicians who had high utilization.

Relationships with purchasers and consumers. The characteristics associated with being "Blue" work to the Plans' advantage in their relationships with purchasers and consumers. The Blues offer purchasers and consumers attractive features, including provider and product choice, access to a valued brand name and national network, and stability. But, as with provider relationships, some of the characteristics that give the Blues their identity work against them, particularly with respect to their ability to change and to innovate.

On balance, the Blues appear to be well positioned, with their broad networks and related availability of PPO and POS products, to offer choice to purchasers and consumers in response to the managed care backlash. While some critics have suggested that the Blues were slow to respond to managed care, the national observers interviewed for this study argued that this has worked to the advantage of the Blues, relative to other managed care companies, as consumer demand has shifted toward less-restrictive managed care products.

As independent local plans, Blue Plan respondents particularly value the BCBSA services that enable them to provide multisite employers and traveling enrollees with access to a nationwide network. While respondents report that the network is not seamless, the Plans and their customers get the benefit of substantial provider discounts in other Plans' markets and central claims processing for national accounts. However, BCBSA does not offer the benefits of standardized national products as do some national managed care companies, with the exception of the Federal Employees Health Benefit product. Regardless of the shortcomings, the respondents thought they have a competitive edge over many national plans because the Blues have coverage in most markets across the United States with sufficient market share to get good discounts.

While these services are important, Plans' number one benefit from BCBSA membership is the local monopoly on use of the trademarks, which was viewed by a number of Plans as their most important asset. Blues respondents widely quoted a marketing study done by the BCBSA that stated that the cross and shield symbols are two of the most widely recognized trademarks in the United States. The Blues believe the trademarks are generally perceived to be associated with good coverage, security, and stability. Several Plans in the study that had stripped "Blue" from their product names have reclaimed it, citing the wide recognition and positive association the name has.

In contrast to the perspectives of most Blue Plan respondents that the trademarks are valuable assets today, vantage respondents across and within each market were more mixed in their assessment of the trademarks' value. In particular, many vantage respondents felt the value of the trademarks across all market segments has been diminishing over time. They did agree with the Blue Plan respondents that the brand names continue to help business in certain traditional segments such as the markets for seniors, individuals, travelers, and unions, but they contended that those lines of business are not profitable in all states. In general, contrary to the claim of respondents at three Blue Plans that purchasers are willing to pay a premium for the trademarks, vantage respondents and national observers suggested that only when the Blues price at market do the trademarks give them an advantage over their competitors.

Respondents reported that the reputation of the brands, along with longevity in local markets, makes the Blues stand out as "stable" and "secure" amid much organizational turnover. Respondents did not expect local Blue Plans to exit the market or be acquired. This stability is an attractive quality to many purchasers who want to ensure the financial viability of their carrier and minimize fallout from administrative and network upheavals. In quite a few sites, the Blues also benefit from the strong preferences of providers and purchasers for local ownership of healthcare organizations, which has restricted the ability of other plans to gain a foothold in the market (Grossman 2000).

While the Blues appear well positioned with respect to purchaser demands, the evidence from this study suggests that this is more a reflection of their legacy—particularly their close relationships with providers and their reluctance to fully embrace restrictive managed care products—than of innovative behavior. In fact, few vantage respondents in any market considered the Blues to be innovative. This is largely tied to their longevity in the market and not-for-profit culture, together with the strong market position they continue to enjoy. The Blues were frequently criticized for being "slow to move," "complacent," and "bureaucratic." In addition, vantage respondents considered them to be "old fashioned" and "behind the times" compared to for-profit managed care companies. One Blue Plan respondent joked that his Plan still worked hard to make sure they never refused a claim, highlighting the tension between indemnity and managed care cultures. Therefore, the common perception that the Blues are an "800-pound gorilla" was not only a reflection of their clout with providers but also a reflection of their unresponsiveness to purchaser demands—for example, to customize products or improve customer service. In a few markets, however, the Blues were praised for being timelier in processing claims and provider payments than were other plans.

Despite the general picture of the Blues as non-innovators, respondents in four markets volunteered specific examples of new products, showing that the Blues can sometimes be innovative. In each case, the Blue Plan was the first to introduce a less-restrictive managed care product in the market, ranging from an open access HMO to a PPO with preventive care benefits. From a national perspective, these products were not new; however, from the perspective of local respondents, the Blues were clearly doing something that had not been done previously in the market, and the Plans and consumers benefited from these introductions.

Strategic Responses of the Blues

Although the Blues continue to be differentiated from their competitors in ways that are beneficial to them and appealing to consumers, they are implementing strategies in response to current market pressures that are diminishing some of the unique benefits they have traditionally provided to consumers. With most Blue Plans no longer subject to regulatory requirements that require them to take hard-to-insure enrollees, their large market share means that they find themselves balancing the demands of being a good corporate citizen against the pressures to enhance margins. Likewise, in the face of increased competition, the Blues are engaging in a significant amount of consolidation and conversion activity that could diminish their local focus and not-for-profit status.

Balancing Profit Margins with Corporate Citizenry

Although most Blue Plans are no longer subject to unique regulatory requirements, Plan respondents felt that the public and regulators still have an *expectation* that the Blues serve the community in ways other plans are not expected to, albeit in more informal and ad hoc ways than in the past. For many Blue Plan respondents, this regulatory legacy is closely linked to the obligation they feel to serve as a good corporate citizen, given their large market share and significant role in the local economy. For those Blue Plans that serve less densely populated areas, the local representation on the Plan's board of directors heightens this pressure. Many Plans were acting to fulfill these expectations by funding local public-health efforts, community events, and civic organizations.

While Blue Plan respondents generally felt it is important to respond to the community's expectations, and, in some cases, it is in fact "good for business" to do so, some respondents suggested that current market conditions require them to carefully balance such demands against the need to maintain margins. For example, several plans noted regulators' expectations that the Blues accept the enrollees from plans that have gone bankrupt. While these Plans have generally complied, one of them said that they now only do so when it is in their financial interest.

The tension between profitability and public benefit is particularly evident in decisions about whether or not to offer products to the hard-to-insure market segments that the Blues have traditionally served, such as the markets for Medicare supplemental insurance (Medigap) and individual coverage. In many sites, Plans—whether nonprofit, mutual, or for-profit—report that they are giving more consideration to profitability when making decisions about offering these lines of business and less consideration to the public benefit role they've played in the past. Arkansas Blue Cross and Blue Shield, for example, continues to offer Medigap and individual products, not because they are required to do so but because they are profitable—so profitable that they are targeted for growth. The opposite is true in Washington, where both Premera Blue Cross and Regence Blue Shield closed their doors to new enrollment in the market for individual coverage. Individual products were very unprofitable in Washington as a result of regulation that restricted premium increases.

Nonetheless, it is not always the case that profitability considerations alone are dictating the Blues' actions with respect to serving hard-to-insure populations. On the contrary, respondents at several Blue Plans report that this is one area in which residual public expectations sometimes affect strategic decisions. In both Michigan and Massachusetts, for example, the Blues continue to offer Medigap at regulated rates they say have caused tens of millions of dollars in losses each year. In Michigan, the Plan is required by law to provide this product. Blue Cross and Blue Shield of Massachusetts is not legally required to sell the product, but as the only in-state plan remaining in the Medigap market, it feels that it is under unique pressure to continue to do so. Although Premera Blue Cross and Regence Blue Shield were able to stop enrolling new individuals in Washington, both were faced with a large amount of public scrutiny and resistance to their actions. While they clearly attracted more scrutiny than other plans that exited because they were the largest providers of individual insurance in the market, the Blues felt they were also subject to lingering expectations of their public benefit role. As one respondent put it, "the Insurance Commissioner is more passionate about the Blues because she perceives them to be a public utility."

Mergers and Conversions Transforming the Blues

Up until 1994, most mergers among the Blues took place within state lines, with the number of Plans decreasing from 110 to 69 between 1982 and 1994. However, with the change in the BCBSA rules at that time allowing investor-owned, for-profit firms, several Plans, including WellPoint Health Networks and Anthem, Inc., saw opportunities to implement geographic-expansion strategies. These moves have set in motion a large number of mergers among Blue Plans across state lines and conversions to mutual or for-profit companies. For the first time, Blue Plans are becoming acquisition targets of out-of-state Plans. Prior to this time, Blue Plans had not merged across state lines and national managed care companies were restricted from acquiring Blue Plans because of BCBSA rules that restricted the ownership share of non-Blues entities in Blue Plans to no more than 5 percent. Together, the mergers and conversions are in the process of substantially altering two unique characteristics of the Blues—local focus and not-for-profit operation—and rendering at least some of the Plans relatively indistinguishable from their for-profit national competitors.

Mergers. Blue Plans that want to expand across state lines typically merge with or acquire other Blue Plans to be able to sell branded products in those new markets. Still the exception rather than the rule, an increasing number of Blue Plans, most notably WellPoint, are engaged in a strategy to acquire non-Blue Plans in multiple markets outside of their licensed service area(s) and to expand enrollment in unbranded products.

The Blues have a number of incentives to expand geographically (Corrigan et al. 1997; Robinson 1999):

1. to gain economies of scale in administration and information systems;
2. to expand products and services;
3. to serve multistate employers;
4. to diversify risk across different market and regulatory environments; and
5. to provide counter-leverage to the consolidation activities of other plans, both Blues and national for-profits.

Mergers also have the potential to enhance access to capital. Capital can be used for further expansions or to finance information systems, product development, or clinical management strategies (Corrigan et al. 1997). Interestingly, one of the most compelling reasons for national plans to merge with or acquire other plans—to increase local market share and improve leverage with providers—is not a driver for the Blues.

A few Blue Plan respondents and national observers expressed skepticism about some of the benefits accruing from merging with other Blue Plans. Some respondents claimed that few economies of scale exist across state lines because insurance products are regulated at the state level, and, in many markets, it is unclear how much business from regional employers has materialized (Grossman 2000). Also, while capital is needed if plans have aggressive acquisition strategies, capital needs to develop tightly managed networks and care management systems have abated because of the managed care backlash and technological advances that reduce the costs of information systems. Many plans already have adequate sources of capital to meet their needs, including reserves and borrowing capacity through for-profit subsidiaries (Cunningham and Cunningham 1997; Robinson 2000).

Despite arguments on the merits, the site visits and activity since then make clear that the Blues are very interested in merging with each other. While at the time of the site visits, regulatory scrutiny and legislation in a number of states had put a damper on merger activity among the Blues across the country, it was still the case that two-thirds of the plans in the study expressed interest in, or had been involved in, merger discussions with other Blue Plans. In fact, two Plans were implementing mergers: (1) BCBS of Central New York joined two other nearby Plans in the state under a nonprofit parent corporation, Excellus, and (2) WellPoint began the process of acquiring BCBS of Georgia, which had already converted to a privately held for-profit company.

More importantly, however, there has been an increase in actual merger activity among the Blues nationally and in the CTS study sites since the site visits. Very soon after the study period ended, Anthem and WellPoint once again began vigorously pursuing Plans across the United States. Most recently, The Regence Group—a nonprofit affiliation of Blue Plans in Washington, other northwest states, and Utah—announced plans to affiliate with the mutual Health Care Service Corporation (HCSC), which operates the Blue Plans in Illinois and Texas as well as other recently acquired Plans.

As Blue Plans continue to consolidate, the national landscape appears to be developing into a tug of war between these three large players— Anthem, WellPoint, and HCSC. While Blue Plans have cited improved efficiency and access to capital as reasons for joining together, recent activity also appears quite rivalrous and reactionary in nature, with these powerful plans and others trying to be the first to pick off the most attractive independent Plans remaining in the market. When Anthem tried, unsuccessfully, to merge with BCBS of Rhode Island in mid-1999, BCBS of Massachusetts was quick to make a counteroffer to acquire or affiliate with the Plan, even though at the time of the site visits, they had no plans to entertain any mergers. Anthem and BCBS of Massachusetts jockeyed over other Plans in New England as well, with Anthem ultimately making three acquisitions. Similarly, when Anthem made an offer to BCBS of Colorado, a number of other Plans, including Wellpoint, HSCS, and Blue Shield of California, made offers as well.

Conversions. The 1994 rule change in the BCBSA was also an important catalyst for conversion activity among the Blues, and they have a number of incentives to do so. As with mergers, access to capital is a key incentive to convert to for-profit status, particularly for plans looking to fund acquisitions. Some plans convert to a mutual or privately held for-profit company to have more operating flexibility than is possible as a nonprofit. For-profit conversions, particularly conversions to publicly offered companies, can provide strong incentives for management to improve operating efficiency. Arguments against conversion also exist. Some Blue Plan CEOs strongly expressed their commitment to maintaining the not-for-profit mission of their Plan. Respondents also noted the challenges of being responsive on a regular basis to public investors in such a low-margin business. Consumer advocates have suggested that the management of plans going public may be driven, in large part, by the opportunities for personal financial benefit (Community Catalyst 1999).

Following the 1994 rule change, Blue Cross of California became the first to convert to for-profit, investor-owned status, setting off conversion activity by other Blue Plans around the country. Many of the early conversion attempts were pursued as a way to gain access to capital markets and to achieve increased flexibility to respond to changing market conditions. However, the frequency with which conversions have been attempted also is closely tied to the merger activity that has been occurring among the Blues. While mergers and conversions do not have to go hand in hand— for example, the formation of non-profit Excellus in New York—the profit status of the merging parties often is not the same. Therefore, amid the recent flurry of mergers, many of the acquired Plans have converted to facilitate the legal process of the merger and align the incentives of all of the parties. So far, only a handful of all Blue Plans have become publicly offered, although many market observers speculate other Plans currently structured as mutual companies or privately held for-profits are poised to go public at some point in the future.

With the prospect that newly formed companies might at some point go public, the recent mergers between Blue Plans, particularly those that involve conversions to mutuals and for-profits, have received a great deal of regulatory and public scrutiny. Given the variation of Plan bylaws and state statutes, every case has transpired differently. Typically, because of the Blues' history as charitable organizations, regulators and consumer advocates want to ensure that a Plan's assets that belong to the public are kept within the state in a nonprofit entity and are not transferred to private investors, Plan executives, policyholders, or out-of-state organizations. Regulators and Plans have wrangled over whether the Plan has ever been a charitable organization under state statutes and, if so, the fair value of the public assets (Consumers Union 2000a). Some states also have proactively proposed or passed legislation prohibiting conversions, requiring regulatory approval, or restricting the movement of assets from a nonprofit into a for-profit parent or subsidiary, as is the case in New Jersey and Washington (Consumers Union 2000a).

This regulatory scrutiny has aborted some merger and conversion attempts and resulted in changes in the terms of others. BCBS of New Jersey had plans to convert to a mutual company to merge with Anthem, but the merger was called off in 1997 when the Plans were ordered to contribute a substantial sum of money to a charitable foundation. More recently, acquiring Plans have begun to offer to donate the full value of the acquired Plan to a charitable foundation as part of the initial terms of the agreement, although assessing the market value of the plan is complex and open to controversy (Consumers Union 2000a).

Mergers and conversions may be scrutinized even if they do not involve the direct transfer of assets to for-profit parents because a variety of other ways exists to transfer assets and structure the new corporate entity that diminish the ability of regulators to scrutinize future activities. For this reason, regulators and consumer advocates in Washington have raised a number of concerns about the recent proposed affiliation between the non-profit Regence Group and mutual company HCSC. First, the affiliation facilitates the transfer of funds out of state. For example, although it is not a full-asset merger, money from the Regence Group's member Plans is to be transferred to a for-profit corporation in Oregon that will provide administrative services to those plans (Consumers Union 2000a). In the event of a conversion, Washington regulators will no longer have an opportunity on behalf of the public to lay claim to those or any other assets moved out of the state. Second, consumer advocates have concern because of the relative ease with which Illinois-based HCSC can convert from a mutual company to a for-profit. Under Illinois state law, HCSC can convert with only a vote of its board of directors. If it decides to do so at some point in the future, Washington regulators will be limited in their ability to scrutinize the conversion (Consumers Union 2000b).

Implications of Strategies for Consumers and Policymakers

As the Blues respond yet again to changing market and regulatory forces, they are making strategic choices that threaten the benefits that consumers have traditionally enjoyed from them. Blue Plans are likely to continue to evolve in ways that make them look more like their national, for-profit competitors, leaving them less accountable and responsive to the demands of local purchasers, consumers, providers, and regulators, particularly expectations about the public benefit role they've traditionally played. As Plans in this study indicated, they are already under pressure to carefully weigh the financial impact of providing community benefit, and, unlike in the past, most no longer have regulatory requirements that put bounds on what they must continue to do. With diminished regulatory requirements, local accountability must work through market and community forces, which are less direct and inconsistent. While some Blue Plans will remain independent, continued consolidation and growth into large regional and national Blues conglomerates is likely. Even informal local accountability is likely to erode somewhat, along with the stability Blue Plans currently offer, as local Blue Plans continue to be acquired by out-of-state Plans. This is particularly true for those Plans that are subject to the demands of Wall Street investors for earnings and growth, which could potentially come at the expense of access and quality.

Consumers could see a net gain from merger and conversion activity if the Blues engage in strategies that support continued local accountability and service, while successfully implementing the aspects of mergers and conversions that are most likely to directly benefit consumers. For example, merging Plans have the option of keeping some functions at the local level to leverage their market presence, such as provider contracting, sales, and customer service, while consolidating others, such as back office operations at the corporate level to leverage economies of scale. For example, BCBS of Central New York, after merging with two other contiguous Plans, continues to do marketing, claims processing, and provider contracting at the plan level, but its product development has been moved to the corporate level. BCBS of Central New York believed that it has benefited significantly from this strategy in being able to rapidly roll out a new POS product that purchasers wanted. In contrast, Anthem was moving toward centralizing many functions, including hospital contracting, in the corporate offices of the Midwest unit. However, in both Indianapolis and Cleveland, Anthem was viewed as an outside plan because its management was in Cincinatti, and purchasers and providers lamented the lack of local focus. At the same time, little evidence was shown in these local markets of the type of care management and quality initiatives for which Anthem had been gaining national attention. After the site visits, Anthem reportedly moved management of BCBS of Indiana back to Indianapolis from Ohio, where it had been moved when Anthem acquired the Plan.

The experience to date of national managed care companies, however, suggests that mergers are difficult and costly to implement, particularly in the short run, and can negatively affect consumers. Companies have benefited from increased access to capital markets to continue their expansion and sometimes, from increased leverage with providers in local markets. These strategies have sometimes generated plan and network instability that have harmed consumers. Slower to materialize have been anticipated outcomes that have the potential to benefit consumers, such as lower costs because of increased efficiencies, improved customer service, more innovative insurance products, and enhanced quality of healthcare (Robinson 1999; Grossman 2000).

State regulators may have options to permit mergers and conversions to move forward while helping to prevent potential adverse effects for consumers. As Blue Plans have pursued mergers and conversions, regulators and consumer advocates have focused on ensuring that public assets remain in-state and are invested for the public good. However, they have also raised concerns about the potential for negative impacts on the affordability of healthcare and local accountability (Community Catalyst 1999). While the terms of mergers and conversions vary significantly, several conversions, including those of BCBS of Illinois and BCBS of Connecticut, require that some portion of the public assets be spent on providing coverage for the underinsured and uninsured (Consumers Union 2000a). In at least one case, state regulators have detailed specific ways in which the acquiring Plan must work to maintain the level of community benefits and local accountability provided by the local Plan. Anthem acquired BCBS of New Hampshire in 1999, agreeing to put the proceeds of the sale into a charitable foundation. In approving the sale, given the dominance of the Blue Plan in that market, the Department of Insurance also imposed 18 conditions on the Plan (Consumers Union 2000a), including a commitment for three years to:

- continue community benefits at the same level of funding to finance such projects as a vaccine program;
- offer a nongroup product;
- maintain a provider network comparable to what had been offered;
- report on complaints to the Department of Insurance;
- maintain employment levels equal to Anthem's employment rates in other states; and
- form a local advisory board to be consulted on any major changes related to the above activities.

This example, however, raises an important question about the appropriate degree of state regulatory scrutiny. Such an approach moves beyond making sure public assets are protected and requires fairly active regulation. It is unclear to what extent other states have the option to, or feel it is appropriate to, impose such requirements on the Blues.

States and the federal government have been moving toward a more level regulatory playing field for insurance regulation, and this principle should generally be applied in regulating the Blues and other sectors in the healthcare industry. This is a particularly critical issue, given the increasing consolidation in both the health plan and provider arenas. For example, recent state-level individual and small group market reforms and managed care regulations have been applied across the board to all firms that participate in the market. Such approaches have the potential to expand the number of individuals who can benefit, while more widely sharing the burden for any costs incurred. Similarly, it is within the regulators' authority to monitor large plans and healthcare providers to ensure that their behavior is not anticompetitive and to oversee conversions of nonprofits to for-profit status. However, such action should be applied consistently to all organizations in the appropriate class (e.g., market share or corporate structure), and the Blues or other healthcare organizations should not be subject to differential treatment unless they also get special benefits from this regulatory treatment.

In general, regulators seem to support this view today. However, they have not always been clear and consistent in letting that decision drive public policy and expectations. In addition, the principle of a level playing field in regulation will not be practical in all instances. The reality is that in some markets, such as New Hampshire and some of our study sites, the Blues are by far the largest health plan, and health plan regulation, de facto, is regulation of the Blues. In addition, as much as the Blues continue to receive tax or other benefits that are of value, they should expect to play a commensurate public-benefit role.

Conclusion

The Blues find themselves at yet another turning point in the evolution of the healthcare market. As the pendulum swings back toward a fee-for-service PPO market, the Blues are well positioned to compete against other managed care companies, given the attractive features they can offer purchasers and their market clout with providers. In almost every market, purchasers and consumers are perceived to value the stability and choice that the Blues offer relative to other plans in an era of managed care backlash and market turmoil. The Blues offer a wide range of products with broad and stable networks. Until recently, in contrast to most other managed care organizations, Blue Plans have remained locally managed, and ownership has not changed hands. Balanced against these strengths are the traditional weaknesses of the "800-pound gorilla," which manifest themselves in a lack of responsiveness to purchasers and providers in some markets and a uniformly poor record on innovation.

However, as the Blues adapt themselves to a changing environment, their transformations may come at a cost. The Blues' strategies today suggest that many of the benefits enjoyed by consumers in the past could erode, leaving the Blues more like their national for-profit competitors. It is possible that changes among the Blues, most notably mergers and conversions, could be structured in such a way as to preserve local accountability. In this respect, regulators can have an important role in ensuring that consumers are appropriately protected. However, the changes occurring among the Blue Plans, as well as in the organization of the healthcare system generally, might also call for a more level playing field where all the relevant entities are subject to the same regulations. As the Blues continue their transformation and as both health plans and providers continue to consolidate, it will be important for regulators to determine what consumer needs are not being met by the market and how to effectively regulate it to improve healthcare affordability, quality, and access.

CHAPTER 4

Specialist Responses to Managed Care

Jon B. Christianson, Ph.D.

Introduction

Through their treatment decisions, specialists historically have controlled a substantial portion of healthcare spending in the United States (Bodenheimer 1999). However, the growth and evolution of managed care has challenged the traditional position of specialists in local healthcare delivery systems (Iglehart 1994). The policies of some managed care organizations (MCOs) have impinged on specialist autonomy (e.g., through treatment protocols) (Sisk 1998; Anders and McGinley 1998); limited access to patients (e.g., through restrictions on network participation) (Guglielmo 1996); reduced fees (Iglehart 1994); and constrained income (the evidence on this point is not clear-cut, however; see Simon and Dorn 1996). Less directly, the relationships that MCOs have forged with hospitals and with primary care physicians have altered the clinical and practice environment for specialists.

In this chapter, we use data from the CTS site visits (Kohn et al. 1997) to identify and describe strategies pursued by specialists to respond to changes in their local market brought about, directly or indirectly, by the growth of managed care. Based on respondent observations in the first round of site visits, as well as documentation in popular press and health services research literature of the intensification of pressures on specialists, we identified the role of specialists in local healthcare markets as a special topic for the second round of visits. The random process used to select

Paul Ginsburg and Cara Lesser provided valuable comments on drafts of this chapter.

sites for the CTS is a strength of this analysis. It ensures that the CTS data provide a cross-section of specialist activity in the United States.

Framework for Discussion

In any local market, three sets of relationships are dominant in determining the practice environment of specialists: two of these relationships—with primary care physicians and hospitals—are longstanding. Specialists have always competed with other specialists for patient referrals from primary care physicians and have depended on these referrals to generate income. Relationships with hospitals are also critical for specialists because hospitals also provide important "inputs"—services and equipment—that specialists use to generate income. The reverse is also true—hospitals depend on specialists to generate hospital revenues.

Prior to the advent of managed care, many, if not most, of the relationships that specialists depended on to provide the inputs—patients, services, and equipment—were informal. In practice, groups of primary care physicians, specialists, and hospitals functioned as "strategic networks," the nomenclature used by economic organization literature (Jarillo and Ricart 1987; Jarillo 1988) and defined as sets of long-term relationships among distinct, but related, organizations for the purpose of gaining or sustaining a competitive advantage in the marketplace.

The growth of managed care over time changed the strategic networks in communities. As MCOs grew, they became large volume buyers of specialty services. Specialists needed to become part of MCO networks to maintain access to patients; this meant entering into formal contractual relationships, which not only determined level of reimbursement but also committed specialists to MCO processes and procedures for forming relationships with primary care physicians and hospitals. For instance, specialists might no longer be able to practice in their preferred hospitals when caring for enrollees of a particular MCO unless those hospitals also were part of the MCO's provider network. Traditional referral relationships with primary care physicians might be disrupted unless the specialists were part of the same MCO physician networks as these primary care physicians. In addition to altering these established strategic networks, MCOs also challenged the traditional autonomy of specialists in the delivery of care to their patients (Brett 1997). Referral limitations, precertification requirements for hospital admissions, drug formularies, and similar measures all intervened in the specialist's day-to-day practice of medicine, altering the "production function" for specialty care.

The rapid growth in number and enrollment in MCOs, and the proliferation of different types of MCO products, created considerable uncertainty in the local market environment for specialists. But, this uncertainty clearly was compounded by the responses of hospitals to MCO growth and resulting declines in admissions. These responses included merging with other hospitals to increase bargaining power with MCOs, purchasing primary care physician practices, and sponsoring physician-hospital organizations as vehicles for contracting with MCOs. All of these activities restructured, to some extent, the historical relationships between hospitals and the specialists on their medical staffs (Jaklevic 1999).

The central objective of the analysis presented in this chapter is to examine the "jockeying for position" (Porter 1998) that has occurred among specialists in response to the growth of managed care in their local markets. Not surprisingly, we found that specialist responses varied considerably across our 12 CTS study sites. This is because at the local-market level, MCO growth has proceeded at different paces and along different paths. In addition, important historical differences exist in the structure of community healthcare systems that also affected the nature of specialist and hospital responses. However, commonalities in specialist responses, which can be understood in the context of "strategic groups," are also likely. Theorists have coined the term "strategic groups" to describe clusters of firms that employ common strategies (Oster 1999) in response to environmental change. Different reasons for strategic groups exist, but ideology sometimes plays a significant role in distinguishing groups.

Specialists can be placed, in a crude sense by their ideologies, into three major strategic groups: (1) academic specialists, (2) specialists who are part of multispecialty groups, and (3) independent specialists. Academic specialists place a high value on research and the application of new technology in patient care, and they are closely tied to major teaching hospitals. Specialists in multispecialty groups value cooperation and collaboration in the organization of services and the delivery of patient care. By virtue of their size and longevity, these multispecialty groups often achieve prominence in their communities, and, as do academic medical centers, they typically are recognized by consumers by their "brand name"—for example, Cleveland Clinic, Mayo Clinic, Virginia Mason. Specialists in unaffiliated single-specialty groups value autonomy and independence. They may practice in one or more hospitals, but they are often identified closely with particular hospitals.

In many, but not all, of the 12 study sites all three strategic groups are prominently represented, but some markets can be characterized by a dominant strategic group. For example, Cleveland is dominated by specialists in large multispecialty group practice and its affiliated or owned hospitals and practices; Boston is dominated by specialists in academic practices; and Phoenix is dominated by specialists in independent, single-specialty practices. However, in many of the study sites, including some with dominant strategic groups, all three types of groups are represented to varying degrees. The idea of strategic groups is helpful in understanding why, within any given market, one might observe an array of different, and sometimes contradictory, specialist responses. Faced with similar environmental changes, specialists in different strategic groups would be expected to respond differently based on their history and shared ideology. Different specialist responses across the 12 study sites can be expected because different strategic groups dominate different sites and the nature and strength of managed care growth varies across sites.

Relationships with MCOs

Two common themes emerged across all study sites concerning current relationships between specialists and MCOs. First, respondents in all sites, except Greenville, shared a perception that there was an oversupply of most, if not all, types of specialists in their communities. (The absence of this perception in Greenville is consistent with secondary data that suggest Greenville had the lowest physician-population ratio among the 12 sites [Trude, West, and McIntosh 1999].) This made it imperative for independent specialists and single-specialty groups, on their own or through participation in networks of providers, to seek out and retain contracts with multiple MCOs. Instances where specialists left an MCO network or refused an MCO contract offer were observed in only three sites, and even in these sites these instances were seen as a rare occurrence. The MCOs used the oversupply of specialists, and the limitations that this placed on specialists' options, to their advantage when negotiating payments with independent specialists; this bargaining power, however, was tempered by the effects of "managed care backlash" (Harris, Ripperger, and Horn 2000). Consumer concerns about quality of care in MCOs and about perceived MCO efforts to manage costs by limiting access to services were reflected in employer negotiations with MCOs. In all of the study sites, respondents reported that consumer demands for large networks and easy access to specialists favored specialists in their negotiations with MCOs. These demands limited the ability of MCOs to exclude specialists, especially brand name multispecialty groups, from their networks and to manage the referral process between primary care physicians and specialists.

While some MCOs' use of capitation approaches to purchase specialty care has received attention in the literature (Defino 1994; Montague 1996), we found that in eight of our 12 study sites the dominant MCO payment method for specialists was fee-for-service, with fees established as a percentage of Medicare fees. Recent declines in fees paid by MCOs were noted by respondents in those eight markets where specialists were paid primarily based on fees. MCOs' focus on securing fee reductions reflected the limited options available to MCOs in controlling specialty care costs, in light of consumer demands for larger networks and easier access to specialty care.

Specialists have attempted to enhance their bargaining positions with MCOs, using approaches that vary by strategic group. For independent specialists, it was imperative that they participated in an organization that aggregates practices for the purpose of contracting with MCOs. A contracting strategy we noted in the first round of CTS visits (in 1996 to 1997)—participation in PHOs—declined in importance over the next two years in seven sites. In many cases, PHOs didn't garner the MCO contracts anticipated by participating physicians, and, in some sites such as Phoenix, they failed financially. On the other hand, in seven of the 12 study sites, physician IPAs, which are typically sponsored by entrepreneurs or hospitals, became or remained important contracting vehicles for independent specialists in their negotiations with MCOs. The growth and significance of IPAs in California have been widely documented (Robinson and Casalino 1995), and we found them to be present and important for specialists in our Orange County site. Typically, specialists' relationships with these organizations are not exclusive. Specialists preferred to participate in multiple IPAs to maximize their access to patients.

It was less common for independent specialists to participate in single-specialty IPAs seeking carve-out contracts with MCOs, although this type of arrangement was noted in Phoenix and Miami. In Phoenix, one entrepreneur helped to establish single-specialty IPAs in cardiology, general surgery, and orthopedic surgery. These IPAs contract with MCOs for a significant number of managed care lives—for instance, the cardiology group serves approximately 175,000 enrollees from one MCO alone. A clear trend toward specialist participation in single-specialty IPAs was not noted in the study sites, as MCOs' acceptance of them appeared limited.

In addition to participating in relatively loosely structured organizations for the purpose of securing MCO enrollees as patients, independent specialists sought to shore up their bargaining positions with MCOs by other means as well. In seven markets, respondents noted a substantial number of mergers among single-specialty groups. For example, in Indianapolis, which has approximately 32 percent more specialists per capita than the national average, mergers occurred in the areas of sports medicine, neurology, urology, obstetrics/gynecology, orthopedics, and urology during the two years between our first and second round of site visits. In addition, two large cardiology groups in Indianapolis merged, creating a combined practice with 87 cardiologists and 52 primary care physicians (Foubister 1999).

Mergers of single-specialty groups do not need to involve large numbers of physicians to enhance specialists' bargaining power. If a merger creates a specialist monopoly in a geographic submarket, it can alter the balance of power in negotiations with MCOs. MCOs that are faced with consumer and employer demands for broad geographic networks to facilitate access to specialty care are hard-pressed not to include these merged entities in their networks.

At the study sites, specialists in the strongest bargaining positions were those able to capitalize either on the sometimes national reputations of their organizations (usually academic medical centers or multispecialty groups) for the delivery of high-quality healthcare or on the unique integrated delivery systems and affiliated provider networks that they had developed over time. In six sites (Boston, Cleveland, Indianapolis, Phoenix, Seattle, and Syracuse), respondents identified specialty organizations that they perceived to offer a differentiated product in the minds of consumers. The strong reputation of these specialty groups translated into a strong and specific demand by employers and consumers to include them in MCO networks. This, in turn, allowed these specialty groups to negotiate contract terms, including payment rates, with MCOs that were more favorable than those terms attainable by independent specialists in the same markets.

Relationships with Hospitals

In most of the study sites, significant merger or acquisition activity among hospitals occurred during the 1990s (Kohn et al. 1997). In seven of the 12 study sites, respondents characterized inpatient care as dominated by a small number of large hospital systems. Hospitals at the study sites generally did not own MCOs with significant enrollments. In fact, the recent sale of hospital-sponsored plans was noted in several study sites. Indianapolis was a clear exception, where a number of the larger MCOs remained under hospital ownership. In five study sites, hospitals continued to sponsor or manage entities (PHOs or IPAs) through which a significant number of specialists contracted with MCOs.

The actual or threatened loss of income as a result of declining MCO payment rates, along with the referral uncertainty created by MCO contracts, led to attempts by specialists to restructure their hospital relationships. For example, independent specialists, a strategic group that experiences considerable pressure from MCO growth, increased their efforts to capture patient revenues that traditionally go to hospitals (for an example of this approach in California, see Ferreter 2000). Specialists in seven study sites were reported to have formed freestanding surgical, and other, facilities either in partnership or in competition with hospitals. A very rapid proliferation of these facilities occurred in some study sites. For instance, in Little Rock, five of the seven freestanding ambulatory surgical facilities have been in operation for less than four years. Of these seven facilities, five are completely physician-owned and two are partially owned by physicians. Cleveland also has experienced very rapid growth in ambulatory surgical centers—from 10 in 1995 to 27 at the time of the site visit—with provider systems being the primary owners of most of these facilities.

A small number of independent specialists pursued an even more ambitious strategy, establishing freestanding specialty hospitals that compete directly with community hospitals. At the time of our site visit, the Arkansas Heart Hospital had recently been established as a joint venture between MedCath—a for-profit company based in North Carolina—and local physicians. These physicians welcomed the MedCath partnership because they perceived that local hospitals were unwilling to purchase desired equipment and allocate the beds needed to support their growing practices. Medicare was the primary source of revenue for Arkansas Heart Hospital because it had not yet negotiated any managed care contracts. In central Phoenix, MedCath entered into a similar arrangement with local heart surgeons, resulting in the construction of the Arizona Heart Hospital near the hospital where these surgeons had previously practiced.

In some instances, specialists used the threat of practicing in freestanding facilities, which would compete with hospitals, to negotiate joint ventures with hospitals (for a description of different types of joint ventures, see Jaklevic 1999). For example, MedCath approached a group of suburban specialists in Phoenix to discuss a joint freestanding heart hospital venture. These specialists used this overture to convince the hospital in which they practiced to form a joint venture with them in constructing a facility dedicated to the care of heart patients.

In other cases, hospitals have successfully resisted specialist pressures for joint ventures. Also in Phoenix, another suburban hospital, which enjoys a more protected geographic market, declined to cosponsor ventures with specialists that would result in the sharing of traditional hospital income streams. Sometimes, hospitals were able to enlist the support of MCOs and employers in resisting specialist efforts. They argued that these facilities were not needed, would duplicate existing capacity, and would therefore raise healthcare costs in the community. In Lansing, a hospital-owned MCO refused to contract with new ambulatory surgery centers, and General Motors supported the MCO's decision. Academic physicians and multispecialty groups in a small number of the study sites pursued strategies involving hospital acquisitions and/or the development of affiliated hospital networks. These strategies are aimed at further enhancing negotiating power with managed care plans or combating the actions of rival groups. For example, at the time of our second round of site visits, the Cleveland Clinic owned 40 percent of hospital beds in Cuyahoga County and 30 percent in the broader six-county primary MSA. In Boston, networks of hospitals have been assembled around competing medical centers and multispecialty groups.

The consolidation of the hospital market at most study sites has created both concerns and opportunities for specialists. Concern about the market power of hospital systems and its potential effect on relationships with specialists is one factor that drives specialists to seek revenue streams independent of hospitals. On the other hand, in some study sites, hospital mergers have led to increased rivalry among the remaining systems, to the benefit of specialists. This is not unexpected. When a relatively small number of similar-sized firms comprise an industry, rivalry among them often is intense (Oster 1999). This description fits the post-consolidation hospital market in many study sites, where hospitals have aggressively recruited specialists in an attempt to offer a complete line of specialty services to MCOs and other potential purchasers. For instance, in Seattle, hospitals were competing against each other for cardiologists and cancer specialists. In Cleveland, the Cleveland Clinic and University Hospitals Health System (UHHS) competed over specialty services. According to some respondents, the Cleveland Clinic is investing heavily in its pediatrics and oncology services, which are both considered historical UHHS strengths. UHHS, on the other hand, is partnering with Southwest General Hospital to develop open-heart surgery, pediatrics, and cancer services, and it is partnering with Lake Hospital for cancer services.

Conclusion

Specialist practice environments clearly are affected by a variety of external forces that are national in scope, such as Medicare reimbursement policies, medical school graduation rates, and demographic trends in the potential patient population. The growth of managed care, and the consolidation of hospitals into larger systems, are two such trends, with impacts on specialists that can vary considerably across local markets. We attempted to track and understand these impacts and specialist responses across our 12 study sites.

Somewhat surprisingly, given that specialists were perceived to be in oversupply at almost all sites, we found numerous instances where specialists were successful in implementing strategies to counteract actual or perceived threats that they associated with MCO growth in their communities; these strategies clearly varied by specialist "strategic group." For instance, many independent specialist practices sought to increase their bargaining power with MCOs through single-specialty practice mergers or by participating in contracting vehicles such as single and multispecialty IPAs. Specialty group mergers at the study sites have largely escaped antitrust scrutiny because they seldom involve a large enough portion of specialists in a geographic market to challenge antitrust guidelines. However, to the degree that specialist practice mergers involve all or most specialists of a given type in a geographic submarket, they can increase the power of specialists in negotiations with MCOs and possibly contribute to premium increases for consumers.

While the merger of specialist practices was a response that we observed at virtually all study sites, the popularity of different types of contracting vehicles varied greatly across sites. For example, single specialty IPAs appeared to be gaining a foothold in Phoenix, but in some sites they were nonexistent. Multispecialty IPAs were most common in Orange County, but even there they were struggling to remain financially solvent. PHOs were present in most sites but appeared to be declining in attractiveness to specialists because they were often seen as primarily serving hospital interests.

Specialists affiliated with multispecialty groups or with academic medical centers typically were viewed by consumers and employers as offering a differentiated, usually desirable, product. They were able to leverage this perception, along with their "brand names," when contracting with MCOs, securing contracts in multiple MCO networks. Many of these specialist-driven organizations also owned or had close affiliations with hospitals.

We also found that independent specialists, in particular, have been successful in developing new sources of income to replace actual or anticipated income losses, which they associated with MCO growth in their communities. Specialists increased their share of revenues traditionally flowing to hospitals by acquiring partial ownership in facilities that produce services historically available only in community hospitals. Ownership of heart hospitals and freestanding surgical facilities, as well as "joint ventures" with hospitals to construct new wings or surgical suites, all could be viewed as attempts by specialists to "integrate backwards" in order to exert greater control over the inputs necessary to produce their services. While actions of this type have been the subject of previous anecdotal reports, we found the current struggle to be intense, quite widespread, and assuming many forms. Interestingly, in some markets the consolidation of hospitals has helped specialists. The larger systems created through consolidation in these markets have competed aggressively for some specialists, in particular cardiologists and surgeons, offering shared ownership of facilities and other partnership arrangements.

CHAPTER 5

Risky Business: The Evolution of Medicaid Managed Care

Lawrence D. Brown, Ph.D.

Introduction

When they resolved to marry managed care and Medicaid in the 1990s, state policymakers, like the hedgehog, knew one big thing: Managed care should slow the rise of Medicaid spending while improving the access to and quality of care Medicaid clients received. As these programs have unfolded, the managed care plans playing in the Medicaid market have discovered, like the fox (Berlin 1993), that success turns on many small things: demographic, strategic, fiscal, regulatory, and other "details" whose individual import and cumulative constraints seldom reveal enough advance clarity to anchor confident planning. The story of Medicaid managed care in the late 1990s was a tale of trials and errors, upbeat entries and unceremonious exits, mysterious collapses, and mid-course corrections, as MCOs struggled to understand the nature of the Medicaid "business" and the range of returns and risks they faced.

Although Medicaid managed care has been sweeping the country, its pace, penetration, and prognosis differ considerably across states and communities. (Managed care arrangements mean "formal enrollment of individuals in a [MCO], contractual agreements between providers and a payer, and some degree of gatekeeping and utilization control performed by a primary care physician, a separate administering arm of the health plan, or both.") (Rowland and Hanson 1996, 150). In the analysis presented in this chapter, such arrangements embrace both managed care "organizations" of diverse pedigree and primary care case management (PCCM) programs.

This analysis uses information from the CTS visits to 12 study sites. In the second round of the site visits (1998–1999), researchers conducted interviews with a cross section of leaders in each community on a range of topics, including Medicaid managed care.

The 12 study sites fall into four general market categories:

1. "Embryonic" markets, typified by Greenville and Little Rock, which are still testing the waters of Medicaid managed care and are still sorting out state strategies and local lineups of players.
2. "Established" markets, typified by Orange County and Phoenix, which are found in states that forcefully committed themselves to Medicaid managed care long ago and have gained extensive, although not always satisfying, experience with it.
3. "Emerging" markets, typified by Cleveland, Indianapolis, Lansing, and Syracuse, which hosted a modest number of managed care plans whose commitment to the Medicaid market and fiscal stability within it remain uncertain in important part as a consequence of fluctuations and hesitations in state policy.
4. "Evolving " markets, typified by Boston, Miami, Northern New Jersey, and Seattle, which witnessed a reasonably steady and substantial growth of Medicaid managed care encouraged by comparatively clear and consistent state policies.

Examining these market categories in light of several important cross-cutting analytical issues—market stability, state policy, access to care, management of care, and consequences for the safety net—is a handy way to distinguish the durable, perhaps intractable, challenges of Medicaid managed care from those that yield more readily to organizational learning over time.

The analysis of the 12 sites presented in this chapter suggests three general propositions. First, the study sites show considerable diversity in market characteristics such as the number and types of MCOs in Medicaid and patterns of entry and exit. Second, the most powerful and pervasive force that shapes these structural differences, and thus the distribution of market types across communities, is state policy, especially payment and regulatory policies. Third, notwithstanding the differences in structures and environments, Medicaid managed care plans face challenges in organizational performance—for instance, "really" managing care—that vary surprisingly (and perhaps disturbingly) little by market type. Market type, in short, may be a distinction that makes little difference for the organizational-performance variables that matter most in Medicaid managed care.

Market Stability

Successful Medicaid managed care presupposes that the Medicaid market will attract the entry and continued participation of enough high-quality MCOs to cover, in time, the vast majority of a state's Medicaid beneficiaries. As might be expected, the validity of this premise varies quite directly with market type. The embryonic market type either relied entirely on PCCM programs, in which providers are paid fee-for-service (Little Rock), or supplemented these with health plans launched by safety net providers—hospitals and clinics that traditionally deliver high volumes of Medicaid services and are anxious not to lose the revenues these services produce (Greenville). Policymakers in Arkansas believed that putting Medicaid beneficiaries into MCOs or paying providers by capitation would antagonize the medical community, diminish the number of providers willing to take Medicaid, and thereby damage access. Physicians in the PCCM program got a monthly $3 per patient fee for such "gatekeeping" as they elected to do, but they faced no financial incentives to manage care.

Respondents contended that policymakers in South Carolina had done little to encourage the growth of Medicaid enrollment in MCOs. For example, beneficiaries could enroll more easily in the PCCM program than in MCOs, providers got higher rates in the former sector than in the latter, and children in fee-for-service Medicaid enjoyed the broad prescription-drug benefits that had once been a distinctive appeal of MCOs. The state's unwillingness to encourage new entrants was matched by the disinclination of for-profit plans to test this unpromising market. Even Community Health Centers (CHCs) responded with understandable lethargy. For them, an interviewee explained, Medicaid managed care meant lower payments up-front plus a delay of several months while the state contemplated adjusting the sum upward to capture more fully the costs of services rendered. In Greenville, the effort to move Medicaid managed care beyond the PCCM model was said to be "stagnating"—an understatement indeed, given that both MCOs in the metropolitan market exited after heavy losses. (Holahan et al. [1998, 63] list South Carolina and Arkansas among the 13 states in which PCCM was the "only type of Medicaid managed care.")

In established markets, by contrast, the practical meaning of Medicaid managed care has come into reasonably clear focus, and improvisation occurs at the edges of a fairly stable cast of organizational characters. Arizona, the last of the 50 states to join the Medicaid program, started with managed care—the Arizona Health Care Cost Containment System (AHCCCS) program—from day one in 1982 (Kaiser 1995; McCall 1997). After several well-chronicled snafus, state managers shaped up AHCCCS into a well-respected Medicaid managed care "prototype" (Fossett 1999).

California, which has long been the state most hospitable to mainstream managed care, launched Prepaid Health Plans in MediCal in 1971, experimented with variations on the theme, and redoubled its efforts to promote MediCal managed care in 1991 (Sparer 1996).

In Orange County, more than three dozen health plans that had participated in MediCal managed care (CalOptima) in 1996 had dwindled to 17, with the active encouragement of state policymakers who believed that confining the right to make competitive bids to plans that had already reached specified minimum Medicaid-enrollment levels enhanced stability and accountability. The Medicaid managed care market in Phoenix was served by six plans, all of pre-1996 vintage. Two plans, one sponsored by Blue Cross, the other by a for-profit company, had left the market since 1996—a development that moved interviewees to expatiate, with the eloquent voice of experience, on the subtle challenges that Medicaid presents to managed care. The Blue Cross plan, noted one interviewee, tried to do too much too fast—for instance, marketing statewide early on only to hit massive problems with its information systems. The exiting for-profit, said another respondent, underestimated the differences between the AHCCCS population and commercial lives: Thirty-five thousand of the former make demands equivalent to 100,000 of the latter. This plan's misadventures triggered a string of rhetorical questions with broad bearing across the 12 study sites: Will a for-profit accept low-to-marginal Medicaid yields? Will it tell the shareholders it could produce no profit on Medicaid in the down years of the insurance cycle? Will it be able to take the negative publicity that Medicaid can bring? These veteran respondent-observers plainly thought not.

Neither in Orange County nor in Phoenix was a dwindling number of participating MCOs viewed as a threat to access. Provider contracts were sufficiently broad and manifold that, as one interviewee put it, if one plan left, patients simply moved to another without changing providers. Policymakers in Arizona and California evidently had confidence that strong, sustained policy leadership had fashioned buyer's markets that struck a decent balance between the virtues of competition and stability.

Emerging and evolving markets are situated in states that, having resolved to promote Medicaid managed care, seek to move beyond discounted fee-for-service PCCM programs and toward a thriving market of risk-bearing MCOs. In emerging markets (Cleveland, Indianapolis, Lansing, and Syracuse), state commitments tend to be more tentative and market responses more limited than in those depicted here as evolving (Boston, Miami, Northern New Jersey, and Seattle).

Where communities fall on this continuum follows from complex interplay between policy stimuli and private calculi. A vigorous Medicaid managed care market presupposes a supply of MCOs sufficient to meet the needs of a growing membership. Defining the demand that evokes that supply is no small task for state policymakers. More MCOs (especially more new, small ones) means more monitoring, more negotiations, and more risk that misrepresentation or underservice by one or a few bad apples will set back the whole effort. State ambivalence—born of multiple goals in partial conflict—creates, in turn, an ambiguous environment for MCOs taking the measure of the Medicaid managed care market. That market—a sizable number of insured lives—is there or getting there, but what patterns of cost and use will it generate? Rates are inviting, or at least bearable, but how long will states that search for savings leave them that way? Regulatory requirements appear to be manageable, but they are also tightening and may continue to do so. A bedrock base of safety-net plans is a natural home for some of this market, but states want to encourage a healthy mix of plan types, including, insofar as possible, commercial plans and traditional nonprofits such as Blue Cross and Kaiser; therefore, entry into the market may look appealing prima facie to an array of plans. All of these variables are matters of more or less, however, and can change quickly. The "value" of these variables and their stability over time largely distinguish emerging from evolving markets.

Policymakers who eagerly will the ends of Medicaid managed care— better access and higher quality at less rapidly rising costs—may not will, or recognize, the means to get there. Respondents in Indianapolis complained that the state allowed far too much freedom to beneficiaries and providers to "flip-flop" between MCOs and the PCCM program, thus impairing the growth of stable panels of enrollees and networks of physicians and, in turn, deterring plans from tackling this market. In Lansing, which was beginning the transition to mandatory enrollment in capitated MCOs in 1997, interviewees grumbled that the state, which added the insult of a steep rate decrease in early 1998 to the injury of serious financial losses by plans in 1997, unwittingly moved plans to reconsider whether this market was an attractive place to linger. Cleveland informants worried that a combination of low state-payment rates and shrinking Medicaid rolls might drive from the market all but safety-net plans that specialize in Medicaid, an anxiety intensified by the departure from Cleveland of a large MCO that tossed 30,000 Medicaid beneficiaries back into the PCCM program while the state negotiated new MCO options for them. In Syracuse, a barren ground for managed care in general (*New York Times* 1999), the Medicaid managed care market, bogged down in disputes over state policies that used competitive bidding to set rates, imposed tough restrictions on marketing and enrollment, and triggered long delays in securing federal approval for the proposed implementation of mandatory enrollment. (Sparer and Brown 1999). As the costs of playing in this market grew clearer and higher, plans began pulling out, ceding business largely to a safety-net plan formed by the city's community health centers.

In the evolving markets, by contrast, rates tended to be viewed as "reasonable," although of course far from munificent, and respondents had little fear that consolidation among plans in the Medicaid managed care market would leave only safety-net plans, good and seasoned soldiers to be sure, but with too little aggregate capacity to serve well a large Medicaid population. The nine Medicaid managed care plans in Miami included a safety-net plan launched by Jackson Memorial Hospital, commercials (one is a large national company that entered Miami in search of Medicare lives and dollars and then took on Medicaid after buying another plan that held this book of business), and one nonprofit plan. Northern New Jersey was rocked by the collapse of the large Health Insurance Plan (HIP), which obliged the state to find new plans for the Medicaid clients among its more than 190,000 subscribers, but a reasonable mix of plans remained, and state regulators were confident that the capacity for high-quality Medicaid managed care was in place. Boston appeared to be the exception that proved the rule: Two of the city's largest MCOs—Blue Cross/Blue Shield and Tufts—left the Medicaid managed care market, which was thenceforth dominated by large MCO number 3—Harvard Pilgrim—in partnership with the Neighborhood Health Plan (NHP), a safety net plan founded by the city's CHCs. Capacity hardly can be said to have shrunk, however: NHP embodied a broad network of well-established CHCs all across Boston and partnership with Harvard Pilgrim—a large MCO whose mission highlights service to all social strata—gave the NHP access to a wide range of providers.

Seattle, on the other hand, shows how strong state leadership may unintentionally (and unluckily) encumber the evolution of Medicaid managed care. Washington inaugurated Medicaid managed care in 1986, made it mandatory in 1993, and achieved a statewide enrollment of about 500,000 (the vast majority of them in MCOs) by 1997. In 1993, however, the state passed a reform package that envisioned eventual enrollment of all state residents in managed care plans and set off a scramble among plans (some novices) for market share. In 1995, much of the controversial reform law was repealed by a legislature newly dominated by conservatives, leaving plans embarked on managed care operations in an "unpredictable and savage market place." (Katz 2000). Within this chaotic context, the state made two policy decisions—(1) to award to the lowest-cost plans the lion's share of auto-assignees, who, the plans protested, generated higher-than-average use and cost; and (2) to require plans bidding for Medicaid business also to participate in the state's Basic Health Plan (BHP) for lower-income people who did not qualify for Medicaid—that forced plans to reassess the stakes of sticking with the Medicaid business. A respondent remarked that "plans in this market change daily" and cited two recent (post 1996) dropouts. In the more dramatic exit, a plan sponsored by a safety-net hospital reconsidered its mission, concluded that it should be providing not insuring care, and "dumped" 60,000 Medicaid and BHP lives to be resettled among the troubled troop of remaining plans. Noting that penetration had not met expectations, an observer cited "declining interest" among plans and providers in Medicaid managed care. Another respondent contended that several plans were pondering a pull out and worried that, barring some sizable shift in state policy, the Medicaid managed care market might, dust having settled, consist only of mission-driven and perhaps solely public plans. Nowhere is it written that evolution cannot be stalled or reversed.

State Policy

Medicaid managed care came into being because state policymakers concluded that the traditional fee-for-service system delivered insufficient value for large Medicaid expenditures. Policymakers differed, however, in their confidence in managed care per se as distinct from market forces more generally, so Medicaid managed care policies understandably varied with the balance of belief and power among state health-policy leaders.

Payments. The policymakers who adopted Medicaid managed care in state after state assumed that they could save money—that is, make state Medicaid spending grow more slowly—as competition induced health plans to deliver Medicaid services more efficiently. A corollary almost everywhere was that states "should" be paying less for Medicaid managed care than they would have been paying under fee-for-service arrangements. How much less and how program payments should be allocated across beneficiaries and plans, however, are questions whose answers varied by state and market type (on the scope of variation, see Holahan et al. 1998).

Payment policies in embryonic markets reflected a diffuse lack of enthusiasm among state policymakers both for the Medicaid program itself and for managed care as "solution" plus a more focused fear that organized medicine would not embrace MCOs. Respondents in Greenville charged that Medicaid managed care payments in South Carolina were so low and slow that they left plans little incentive to enter the market. Little Rock informants recounted that Arkansas policymakers mainly brandished the prospect of MCOs as a threat to induce physicians to participate in the PCCM program. Unwilling to raise payment rates over the last four years, policymakers sweetened their offer by speeding up the processing and payment of claims.

As might be expected, attitudes and issues surrounding payment were quite different in the established market sites, which reflected long years of political accommodation between policymakers and plans. In Orange County and Phoenix, rates were, as an Orange County respondent put it, "ok but flat." Interviewees in both sites underscored, however, that in payment policy practice does not make perfect: Once comfortably beyond the basics that bedevil payments in such sites as Greenville and Little Rock, established markets find a rich array of subtle challenges. Arizona and California, for example, were widely characterized as too slow to adjust rates upward to reflect new and better information about the differential risks and costs of plan enrollees. In both sites, " carve outs"—retaining fee-for-service payments for certain services that allegedly do not lend themselves readily to capitation—were controversial. Phoenix observers, for instance, applauded the return of dental services to fee-for-service because doing so increased the number of participating dentists, but they deplored the exclusion of behavioral healthcare from the managed care program because (said they) the results were badly underfunded programs, long waiting lists, inadequate drug rehabilitation, and general chaos.

Plans in both sites were said to be losing money on Medicaid managed care in the last year or two, but interviewees generally noted that state-payment policies were not the sole or main cause. Characteristics of beneficiaries, dwindling Medicaid rolls as a result of strong regional economies and welfare reform, and insurance cycle vagaries also played their part. In Arizona and California, as in their ten tracked counterparts, rate policies were perpetually "under review" in the state capitals by budget makers; health-policy specialists (executive and legislative); actuaries; consultants; and organizations of plans, providers, and advocates.

Perceptions of payment in the four emerging markets closely parallel, and of course help explain, the bipolar pattern of entry and exit sketched above. Indianapolis interviewees contended that the state set payments too low to trigger much interest in this market and used old data and inadequate measures of risk to boot. Respondents in Lansing, Cleveland, and Syracuse worried that sharp rate cuts might drive plans from the market. The general message was that state policymakers were demanding from Medicaid managed care larger, quicker savings than market realities could deliver.

The evolving markets are a different story. Informants in Boston noted that state policy did reasonably well by the city's Medicaid managed care plans, largely because Massachusetts adjusted rates generously to account for members' risks. (Rates distinguished among welfare recipients, the severely disabled, people with AIDS, SSI clients, and those dually eligible for Medicare and Medicaid [Holahan et al. 1998, 57]). Miami respondents mildly regretted the decline of Florida's capitation rates from 95 to 92 percent of fee-for-service payments, but none portrayed a market in grave peril as a consequence. Plan officials and state policymakers in Northern New Jersey generally agreed that the state was subordinating the drive for deep savings to its hopes of developing a market with an adequate census of good-quality plans. These three states seemed to have a longer time horizon than their four "emerging" counterparts and to be more reconciled to deferring the short-term gratification of savings in Medicaid until markets had been carefully built. (Seattle stood out from this pack because Washington's rules for participation in Medicaid managed care posed unusual complications for estimations of cost and adequacy of payments.)

Enrollment. States shape Medicaid managed care markets by setting rules of conduct as well as rates of payment. Among the most important regulations are those defining how plans market to and enroll Medicaid beneficiaries. One of the signal virtues of Medicaid managed care is supposedly the empowerment it confers on beneficiaries to choose, from among a range of plans, those that best meet their needs; therefore, such functions as furnishing accurate factual information and interpretations and answering beneficiaries' questions are central to a well-working market. Policymakers in most states have come to suspect (or, in such cases as New York and Florida, learned directly from bad experience) that leaving marketing and enrollment to plans themselves invites misrepresentation by enrollment agents who are eager to boost the plan's market share and their own commissions, and cherry picking by plans that want to dodge bad health risks. Thus, most states either start with or turn to an enrollment broker chosen by and under contract to the state itself to do these vital jobs. Predictably, the main exceptions in the study sites were the embryonic markets. In Little Rock beneficiaries stayed with or changed to physicians participating in the PCCM program, which is not deemed to need brokering. Greenville respondents noted that South Carolina had junked plans for an enrollment broker and instead entrusted enrollment to the understaffed and hectic state Department of Health and Human Services, which allegedly was in no hurry to promote Medicaid MCOs.

Enrollment brokers got high marks from the sites that used them for averting overt misrepresentation and cherry picking, but the processes by which beneficiaries get and use information in their enrollment decisions remained obscure and frustrating to respondents in all market types. Telling beneficiaries what they "need to know" and ensuring that they understand what they have heard or read are tough tasks that entail communicating complex information to consumers who may lack phones, addresses, basic literacy, or legal residency and who may have given little thought to the tradeoffs among multiple criteria that choice of plan entails. Almost universally, interviewees lamented that many beneficiaries enter managed care with woefully little grasp of its fundamentals—the need to pick a plan, select and visit a primary care physician (PCP) for an examination, call the PCP before setting out for the emergency room, among others. No less widespread was the sense that the realm of consumer "education" was basically a black box—who ought to be saying what to whom, and how much disappointment with the giving and using of information lay with beneficiaries as distinct from "educators" or the process itself—were recognized as crucial questions to which good answers remained largely undiscovered.

Amid the intangible and hard-to-measure nuances of consumer psychology and choice, one numerical indicator—the rates at which enrollees fail to choose a health plan and are therefore "auto-assigned" to one by the state or its broker—offers crude but suggestive commentary on the adequacy of education at the point of enrollment. A reasonable a priori prediction—the more "evolved" the market, the better the educational techniques in place and so the lower the rates of auto-assignment—did not hold up. Informants estimated auto-assignment rates in Phoenix and Orange County to be at 30 to 40 percent and 25 to 30 percent, respectively, whereas in Northern New Jersey, a less established site, the rate ran at only about 10 percent. (On variations in approach in a different sample of states see Holahan et al. 1998, 48–49 and 62).

Low auto-assignment rates are understandably prized as a sign that informed consumer choice is alive and well and that affiliation of consumers with "wrong" plans is minimal, but forcing these rates downward is no simple matter. Informing consumers—and still more, educating them—are labor intensive, costly endeavors, and the opportunity costs of dollars thus spent are vexing even to states determined to do enrollment "right." Clearly the informational difficulties most sites continue to confront, the failure of these difficulties to yield to market maturity and experience, and the unexpected success in evolving sites such as Northern New Jersey offer abundant evidence and rich variations on the theme of informational "empowerment" of low-income consumers.

Reporting. State regulators not only try to help Medicaid beneficiaries choose the right plan but also require plans to collect, analyze, and submit data on a wide range of performance measures, which presumably show how well they treat beneficiaries once enrolled. States tend to start by demanding fairly basic data—number of immunizations given, number of primary care encounters, and so on—and then expand the scope of reporting as federal overseers, managed care specialists in the state health and insurance bureaucracies, Medicaid advocates, and media investigators raise questions that plans must answer.

Everyone interviewed on the matter agreed that such reporting requirements are needed both to protect beneficiaries and to prod plans and providers toward improvements in quality. Most, however, also concurred that states tend to multiply reporting demands but pay too little attention to the feasibility and cost of compliance and the usefulness of what is transmitted. The medical director of a Miami plan, for example, summarized the implications of a series of seemingly small demands for data. In the "old" days (said he) a medical director satisfied the requisites of quality reporting by sitting down to type out a few lines on how physicians were reviewed. Now, by contrast, quality is monitored by scientific "studies" that scrutinize not only processes of care for specified conditions but also their outcomes. Experts on research design and biostatistics must be brought on staff; sizable bodies of data must be recorded, "cleaned," and analyzed; and management information systems adequate to these analytic tasks must be put in place. These steps take time, money, and personnel, which resources, of course, are beset by other growing managerial demands. These efforts to monitor and enhance quality are unobjectionable in the abstract, but in practice regulations accumulate from myriad and uncoordinated sources: the federal Health Care Financing Administration, the states' general framework of managed care rules, their tomes of constraints targeted on Medicaid managed care in particular, and the standards promulgated by accrediting bodies such as the National Committee for Quality Assurance.

As with marketing and enrollment rules, one might suppose that established sites would cope with compliance more smoothly than less "advanced" sites and, as in that case, one would be wrong. Orange County respondents, for example, sang a refrain that echoed across all 12 sites: The state lacked adequate basic data on simple measures such as the number of Medicaid managed care beneficiaries who got screenings and other services. Encounter data were flawed because, the state contended, providers failed to collect the necessary numbers and forward them to Sacramento in a usable format. Providers rejoined that state-reporting requirements were too vague and too costly. The state was, of course, working on these problems and considering innovative strategies such as paying a bonus to plans that did well with their data. Interviewees across the study sites agreed too that this paucity of good data, properly packaged and analyzed, interferes mightily with the feeding back of performance findings, which is widely viewed as indispensable not only to improvements in providers' work but also to the education of informed consumers choosing among health plans.

Access to Care

Data limitations notwithstanding, respondents in the vast majority of sites agreed that Medicaid managed care had markedly improved access to care, at least in the quite particular sense of an increased number of providers willing to take Medicaid patients (see, however, Lillie-Blanton and Lyons 1998). The sole, and predictable, exceptions were the embryonic markets. An interviewee in Greenville flatly declared that as yet South Carolina physicians were not much interested in Medicaid, let alone Medicaid managed care. The readiness of Little Rock physicians to participate in Medicaid was said to be contingent on the state's refusal to push MCOs and capitation or otherwise to pressure the PCCM gatekeepers to manage care.

At the other extreme, respondents in the established markets agreed that state policy had, in essence, made of Medicaid managed care an opportunity few providers could refuse. In both Orange County and Phoenix, interviewees explained that so many physicians and hospitals were in so many Medicaid managed care plans that the inevitable movement of providers in and out of plans for financial or other reasons had little adverse impact on enrollees. Informants emphasized that these gains extended to specialists as well as PCPs. (An Orange County observer remarked on a specialty group that had begun building its own primary care capacity in order to play better in this market.) In Orange County and Phoenix, more providers wanted to participate in Medicaid managed care than the states cared to accommodate—a prominent contrast with the embryonic markets.

Informants in the emerging and evolving markets were not yet fully convinced that Medicaid managed care had become a buyer's market, but they voiced pleasant surprise at the readiness of providers to get with the program. The ranks of PCPs seeing Medicaid patients have grown. Specialists may regard Medicaid managed care as, in the words of one interviewee, "lots of paperwork for little money;" not all beneficiaries found ready access (the "undocumented woman with abnormal paps" was a problematic case in point, said one informant) and some specialists—gynecologists; ear, nose, and throat physicians; and orthopedists were sometimes cited—stayed in short supply. On the whole, however, managed care had expanded access to specialty care for Medicaid beneficiaries, and, as one respondent asserted, "hospitals that wouldn't contract with these plans do so now." Rough edges remained—for instance, informants in Indianapolis groused that the state's decision to contract with no more than two MCOs in each major region obliged competitors to stretch their networks too thinly across large, often largely rural, areas. All the same, improvements in formal access seemed to be a clear and near-ubiquitous victory for Medicaid managed care. Evidently, in the face of fairly firm state commitments to this enterprise, few providers chose to play chicken and run the financial risk of loitering too long on the outside looking in.

Management of Care

Although understandably pleased with the enlarged provider networks and enhanced consumer choices Medicaid managed care had wrought, respondents in all 12 study sites warned that the mechanics and dynamics that govern the delivery and management of care cannot be summarily inferred from the formalities of access. Making care available and managing it are two different matters, and interviewees voiced considerable skepticism that Medicaid managed care was scoring impressive victories on the latter count. As troubling as the omnipresence of misgivings about care management across the sites, moreover, was the absence of evidence that these processes improve with the maturation of Medicaid managed care markets.

Interviewees in all four market types identified barriers—pretty much the same barriers across sites and market types—to care management that are stubborn and perhaps intractable. First, respondents complained that Medicaid beneficiaries enter managed care plans with too little information about how to capitalize on the system's advantages and how to navigate its channels of access. An observer in Greenville lamented that Medicaid managed care enrollees, like the Medicaid population in general, shuttled back and forth between CHCs and hospital residency clinics, were disinclined to stick with one doctor, and dropped into ERs whenever they pleased. At the other end of the market continuum, an Orange County respondent remarked that reminders failed to move many new Medicaid managed care members to get a health assessment within four months of joining the plan, as recommended. According to an interviewee in Phoenix, AHCCCS providers complained of no-show rates for appointments that sometimes reached 40 percent. Even in that seasoned and savvy program, observers contended that such basic skills as making and keeping appointments and avoiding no-shows, walk-ins, and drop-ins to the ER eluded many beneficiaries. The obvious solution to these problems—fuller, better education up-front and over time—is easy to articulate but tough to implement. For one thing, as a Lansing respondent noted plaintively, it is hard to "identify what to educate them on." For another, wide-ranging and sustained educational outreach is labor intensive, costly, and slow to show results in health or financial outcomes.

Second, plans have trouble managing care, and educating subscribers, because they are often ill-prepared for the medical and social challenges they face. An interviewee in Indianapolis explained that the state "thought that this population [women and children] were basically healthy, but that's not so. There are lots of chronic illnesses, and care management services are not in place. We need more identification of special need populations and patient conditions... "and (of course) more education." Medicaid managed care would work, urged a Miami respondent, if "instead of ignoring the social aspect of care delivery, it were designed according to the condition of the poor." Such "designs" are a long organizational stretch for many MCOs, however.

Third, discontinuities endemic to Medicaid itself often defeat plans' attempts to learn from experience and go far to explain why established and evolving markets reprised so many of the managerial frustrations of their less-advanced counterparts. When changes in employment, family, residency, or other status render beneficiaries ineligible for Medicaid, they are obviously no longer eligible for Medicaid managed care and are disenrolled from their health plan. Each month brings Medicaid managed care plans long printouts of new and former members. A Phoenix respondent conjectured that this churning may plague Medicaid managed care plans with snowballing adverse selection. Strong regional economic conditions, plus federal welfare reform, move healthier beneficiaries off Medicaid and into low-paid private sector jobs that seldom offer health insurance. When hard economic or personal times hit, the ex-beneficiaries return to Medicaid, and to managed care, with accumulated medical needs that have, for want of coverage, gone untreated and now register as powerful pent-up demand for services they are newly at "leisure" to pursue. Meanwhile the most "continuous" beneficiaries are the least employable—a condition that is sometimes a proxy for poor health, behavioral problems, or other indicators of high maintenance, high-cost cases. In essence, the logic of Medicaid enrollment decrees that Medicaid managed care plans cannot win: They are asked to achieve savings by managing the care of a membership mix that grows steadily sicker, more costly, and harder to manage effectively, much less efficiently.

Cyclical theory aside, plan respondents asserted almost universally that discontinuities in eligibility interfere drastically with agendas for educating beneficiaries and managing their conditions. Many enrollees were simply not with the plan, or the program, long enough for "comprehensive, coordinated, continuous" care to kick in and do much good. As Gold (1999, 1646) remarks, "high levels of eligibility turnover... are inconsistent with the managed care model." Whether foreknowledge of this problem deters care management is an important but touchy question. If plans perceive that the benefits of their excursions into care management are realized, if at all, by "the community"—institutions that serve newly uninsured workers, private health plans, or other MCOs—these activities may be a collective good whose benefits particular plans cannot dependably appropriate and which they therefore have no monetary incentive to supply—a bit of an embarrassment for the traditional theory of "health maintenance" organizations.

Not surprisingly, no interviewees averred that Medicaid managed care plans in their community followed this economic logic to its pitiless conclusion. The issue, however, is not yes or no but more or less. A respondent in a large commercial plan in Miami observed that a MCO can do well financially in Medicaid managed care by signing up large numbers of beneficiaries—many of whom tend, at least initially, to be low users of care—and collecting the monthly capitation sums per member per month. The lines that separate "expecting" service use to stay low, "hoping" that it does, and delivering "too few" services are fuzzy both for plans that work with fluid enrollment rolls, inadequate data, and tough competitive pressures and for regulators who view plans at a distance. How rational then is it for plans in vigorous competitive markets to go the extra mile—to make the sizable investments in staff, time, information systems, and outreach needed to advance "true" management of care? This issue, a source of anguish both economic and philosophical, is much on the minds, although seldom on the lips, of those who manage and regulate Medicaid managed care plans.

Consequences for the Safety Net

Most Medicaid managed care sites are less than fully "established," and even Orange County and Phoenix have not worked out all the bugs in this challenging fusion of policy and markets. As the 1990s ended, Medicaid managed care remained an experiment that could fail or falter. Because the verdict is far from final, the unfolding of Medicaid managed care is of more than casual concern to so-called safety-net institutions—clinics and hospitals, usually public or nonprofit, that cared for Medicaid beneficiaries and the uninsured before managed care made the former population more profitable and could be left holding the bag if Medicaid managed care does not wear well. A key policy question, then, asks what Medicaid managed care is doing to, or for, the safety net (see Cunningham et al. 1999a and 1999b; Grogan and Gusmano 1999; Lipson 1997).

Safety-net providers play in the Medicaid managed care market because their fear of being discarded in competition outweighs their fear that managed care revenues will pay them less, maybe much less, than Medicaid fee for service. Luckily, these providers and the plans they may form do not live by Medicaid alone. As they struggle to cut costs and improve marketing, they also draw funds from the State Children's Health Insurance Program (SCHIP), Disproportionate Share Hospital payments (DSH), Medicare, and more. But they also worry about the implications of welfare reform and unpleasant surprises in annual federal budget acts, hoping that as it all sorts out they can stay afloat financially. In this context, Medicaid managed care may not be a make-or-break variable, but it is generally more than marginal. And it gains prominence insofar as commercial and other nonsafety-net plans decline to enter problematic markets or test them and then withdraw—trends visible in many sites in the sample. Some observers worry that after suffering the effects of transitory competition from bird-of-passage MCOs, weakened safety-net institutions and plans will resume their roles as providers and insurers of first and last resort for both the Medicaid population and the uninsured.

The established markets illustrate well the perils of laissez faire competition for the safety net and the policy options for addressing them. AHCCCS is big business for Phoenix CHCs, all of which contracted with the program. Members of the state's Association of CHCs were said to have 20 percent of AHCCCS enrollees in Maricopa County; these enrollees accounted for 40-50 percent of CHC revenues on average. An interviewee explained that the Arizona Physicians IPA contracted willingly with the CHCs because doing so made good business sense: "They're in the community, they know the population, they're accepted, they're good people." To revenues from Medicaid managed care, SCHIP, and other accustomed sources, CHCs added funds from a tobacco tax (legislation governing the distribution of which the Association of CHCs helped to draft) enacted in 1995. Arizona conservatives, an informant observed, value CHCs as a "nongovernmental alternative."

Not all of Phoenix's safety-net providers fared as well under Medicaid managed care as did the CHCs, however. A respondent at the Indian Health Service (IHS) contended that it was losing patients to managed care plans. The county's only safety-net hospital, which is a major Medicaid provider, wanted to boost its AHCCCS business beyond the 10 to 12 percent market share it then enjoyed. Public health activists contended that Medicaid managed care had been hard on the county health department, whose own plan suffered an enrollment drop and adverse selection as Medicaid managed care enrollees sought greener pastures. Moreover, charged these critics, the MCOs were too quick to urge enrollees to visit the health department for services for which the plans then declined to pay. In the skeptics' eyes, CHCs waxed under Medicaid managed care while the rest of the safety net waned.

In Orange County, Medicaid managed care seemed to be no less worrisome for the public health safety net, more problematic for the CHCs, but more proactive in putting a safety net under the safety net. Notwithstanding state requirements that plans try to contract with "traditional providers" in Medicaid, Orange County CHCs lost market share. (Bindman et al. [2000] argue that problems in California's safety net stem more from declining MediCal rolls than from the growth of managed care in the program.) Given a choice, a respondent explained, beneficiaries often forsake safety-net providers that have indeed always been there for the poor but are not viewed as especially consumer-friendly. The state's attempts to redress the balance by favoring safety-net plans in auto-assignments were controversial. One respondent summarized the tough questions: "Should [safety-net providers] be allowed to suffer as clients vote with their feet? What if they're teaching hospitals with critical functions? Or public hospitals with lots of indigent patients?" As these disputes ground on, MCOs geared up to the play the game—that is, win a "safety net" designation—and thus enhanced market share by means of auto-assignments. Meanwhile, interviewees remarked that safety-net clinics were spending more time and resources on strategic plans, new buildings, staff training, patient education, and public relations in hopes of competing better and stemming financial losses.

In the four emerging markets, respondents contended that state payment levels were too low either to attract and retain many nontraditional providers in the Medicaid managed care market or to cover the costs of safety-net providers and plans that cannot easily exit. In Miami, by contrast, earmarked public trust funds managed by a special public authority sustained Jackson Memorial Hospital and, in some measure, its Medicaid managed care plan. Risk-sensitive rate-setting measures in Massachusetts helped Boston's broad and well-settled CHCs stay solvent, as too, of course, did their partnership in the NHP with the mission-minded Harvard Pilgrim plan. State payments widely perceived as reasonable in New Jersey also worked to the advantage of safety-net providers in Northern New Jersey communities. (In Seattle, by characteristic contrast, safety-net providers feared that when or if the chaotic market settled down, they would be left with the lion's share of bad risks and high costs.) Evidently, states and counties can assist the safety net in many different ways. The one constant is that it cannot be expected simply to take care of itself in the intensified competition for its traditional clients.

Conclusion: What Do Markets Mean for Medicaid?

A Seattle interviewee neatly summarized the unfolding institutional dynamics in this and the other tracked sites: "The system is becoming more focused on what it means to be in this business, and not just in terms of efficiencies in patient services." Meanings remain very much in the making.

Medicaid became a subsidiary of the managed care "business" as part of a larger intellectual shift in health policy. The first session of a Health Economics 101 course formerly taught that healthcare was not and could not be a normal market—indeed that it was one big exception to the "laws" that governed much of the rest of the economy. Over the last 20 years, a radical challenge to this view has taken hold in some influential intellectual quarters: Healthcare can be and should be made to behave like other industrial sectors. One needs only to do it right: Get purchasers organized; give them data that inform careful choices among competing health plans; make competition among plans trigger new efficiencies among providers, and so forth, down a normalizing checklist, which, if successfully applied, makes the producing and buying of health services little different in principle from the producing and buying of, say, toasters.

As the CTS indicates, however, "doing it right" is no simple job, involving as it does not mere savings and production efficiencies but also the proclaimed protection and enhancement of access and quality of care. Medicaid managed care programs must proceed within a framework that honors the multiple goals that public policy assigns to the enterprise. That framework starts with governmental rules—partly national, mainly state. State decisions on overall payment rates, nuances such as risk adjustments to those payments, allowable marketing and enrollment practices, and reporting requirements (to name the most salient regulatory arenas) set the boundaries of the Medicaid managed care business. These decisions vary with the political philosophies that guide state policy over time, and these variations in turn encourage differentiations in market type, captured here in the continuum of four market categories.

Within these market types, health plans ponder comparative advantage—their comparative advantage in entering the Medicaid market and the comparative advantage of that market in their larger product mix. Commercial plans or large national nonprofit MCOs participate in Medicaid when the commanding market share they seek argues for a mixed portfolio and Medicaid appears to be too promising an addition to cede a priori to competitors. Big Medicaid enrollments can yield attractive capitation revenues—an appealing business proposition so long as use of services stays low or moderate, payment rates remain high "enough," and regulatory impositions are tolerable. Even when the big ifs cooperate, however, these plans often find it easier to take on Medicaid than to do well by and with the program. Their decisions about entry and exit are largely if not purely opportunistic. If they can make money on Medicaid managed care without undue aggravation, they come and stay. If returns are negative (or too low, or too cumbersome administratively, or accompanied by too much doubt-ful publicity), they defer or leave (McCue et al. 1999).

For safety-net providers and the plans they sometimes sponsor, success in or with Medicaid managed care is critical to retaining a key part of their core business. Contracting with commercial plans on favorable terms and launching safety-net plans and keeping them afloat are not simple tasks, however. Commercials may put safety-net providers on their panels for symbolic reasons but direct the lion's share of referrals to more "efficient" caregivers. Shouldering risk and health insurance functions are new and tough challenges for many safety-net institutions that seek to form their own plans (Sparer and Brown 2000), and the well-advertised presence of newly available alternatives to these traditional Medicaid sites may invite beneficiaries to go elsewhere. Moreover, the comparative advantage, or ne-cessity, of riding the waves of Medicaid managed care depends partly on how providers and plans are faring with such additional public payment sources as SCHIP, DSH, and Medicare. Safety-net plans in general prefer "voice" (especially if state policymakers are attentive and responsive listen-ers) to the exit option, but the latter is seldom out of the question. Opti-mists hope that Medicaid managed care has brought new plans and pro-viders to the program's beneficiaries and that the enhanced access they ensure will endure. Pessimists fear that the pressures of the bad business climate state policymakers may unwittingly, or indifferently, produce will in time compel Medicaid managed care to collapse into a cadre of usual-suspect providers, treating the usual patients with less money and not insignificant residual damage sustained from the experiment itself. A rough guess from an inspection of the 12 study sites is that each camp may prove right in half the cases.

State policy and calculations of comparative advantage in specific mar-kets are key defining features of the Medicaid managed care business, but they are not the only ones. The raw materials for the production functions of this business are the populations serviced. As PCCM programs yield to "real" managed care and MCOs, plans contemplating the Medicaid market must decide whether to accept a proffered or bargained capitation sum per member per month and endure along with it all or some of the risk of pro-viding a broad range of health services to beneficiaries on their rolls. The basic business decision—to enter or pass on the Medicaid managed care market and, once in, to stay or go—turns critically on how plans assess the needs and demands of the Medicaid population and the costs of meeting them. In 1999, these computations still entailed abundant decision mak-ing under uncertainty. Some plans were ill-equipped to cope because they lacked experience, good information systems, or managerial acumen. Even those that knew the score, however, often found that serving the population "well," as defined by the theoretical promise of managed care, was a herculean calling.

Unlike the variables of state policy and comparative market advantage, these issues seemed to differ disturbingly little over time and across the study sites. The litany and its lingo—consumer education, appropriate use and site of services, outreach, case and care management, continuity, and other muscles and sinews of "real" managed care—lingered on, pointing to a vision largely unrealized. Part of the problem turned on organizational learning: Medical providers and health plans were slow to recognize the crucially nonclinical character of much care management in Medicaid. Activities such as persuading enrollees to choose a plan and PCP, gathering information on health status, getting people in for immunizations and examinations, monitoring chronic conditions, and ensuring that members take medications demanded sophisticated and timely interventions by a sizable corps of well-trained community personnel, social and mental health workers, home health workers, nutritionists, and other "outreachers." Mounting such interventions cost-effectively, which is hard enough for stable populations, makes vast managerial demands when the population in question churns on and off Medicaid and in and out of Medicaid MCOs. How much stability among customers does genuine "management"—of medical care or more mundane products—presuppose?

Presumably experience brings usable knowledge, and somewhere along the learning curves these conundrums yield to reliable categories in plans' management information systems and thus become grist for some semblance of planning and management. Many, maybe most, plans have a good way to go, however, leaving many managers and observers wondering how good a job they can afford to do for Medicaid clients and for how long.

Policymakers moved to Medicaid managed care because they bought the big idea that the healthy incentives of MCOs in a competitive milieu would channel wasted healthcare dollars into better medical care. Fuller understanding of the many small details that collectively constitute the practical challenges of Medicaid managed care suggests, however, that "real" managed care for the Medicaid population will deliver few budget savings and may well consume existing and "wasted" program dollars and plenty more. If so, the initial intellectual public offerings that put Medicaid in the managed care business would seem to need fresh conceptual capital.

CHAPTER 6

Anticipated Reactions, Uncommon Denominators: The Political Construction of Managed Care Regulation

Lawrence D. Brown, Ph.D.

"A newspaper... accepts as truth anything that is plausible. We start from that assumption."

Honore de Balzac, *Lost Illusions*, p. 350

Then Mr. M'Choakumchild said... "This schoolroom is an immense town, and in it there are a million of inhabitants, and only five-and twenty are starved to death in the streets, in the course of a year. What is your remark on that proportion?" And my remark was... that I thought it must be just as hard upon those who were starved, whether the others were a million, or a million million. And that was wrong, too.

Charles Dickens, *Hard Times*, p. 75

Introduction

Even mild acquaintance with the American mass media suggests that the latter-day dominance of managed care has been a disaster mitigated only by cost considerations (in which case, critics might allow it to rise to the level of Pyhrric victory). Newspaper and television reports routinely record "abuses" inflicted on innocent patients by greedy MCOs and complement the bad daily news with extended exposes of this "profit-hungry industry." The mere mention of managed care in movie soliloquies, television monologues, radio diatribes, and political cartoons moves viewers and listeners to laughter and tears (Peterson 1999). The media and their messages convey a palpable sense of loss of better olden days; of a once-trusted healthcare system gone bad; of the replacement within that system; of providers and managers who had "a special inaptitude for any kind of sharp practice" (Dickens 1998, 46) with sharpies and frauds.

Political leaders caught the popular drift and got on the case. State legislators have busily enacted patient bills of rights and protection laws of varying length and stringency (by one count, more than 600 regulatory bills were introduced in the states between 1996 and 1998). Meanwhile some 50 patient-protection measures were introduced in the 105th Congress, and by February 1999 more than ten "comprehensive" managed care reform bills were before the 106th Congress (Marsteller and Bovberg 1999, 1).

Those who contemplate healthcare systems within the serene groves of academe are often at a loss to account for the unpleasantness (for a wide-ranging set of accounts see *Journal of Health Politics, Policy and Law* 1999). Opinion surveys regularly report that members of MCOs enjoy quite high levels of satisfaction with their health plans and healthcare (note, however, Jacob's and Shapiro's [1999, 1025] discussion of a "striking" downturn in the public's assessment of the "quality of treatment under managed care as it has expanded."), and a sizable, albeit far from conclusive, literature finds "few consistent differences" in the quality of care rendered by MCOs and traditional arrangements and "generally equivalent outcomes" among HMO and conventional insurance enrollees (Glied 2000, 739). Evidently, consumer ratings—"the average experience of those who use a service"— and public opinion, which reflects "people's own experience" plus that of family and friends "as day-to-day consumers of care," have moved out of sync (Blendon et al. 1998, 90). California fittingly captures the paradox: A survey of members of HMOs, IPAs, and PPOs in that state found that "most people were satisfied or very satisfied with their health plan," but between 1990 and 1997, the state legislature passed 89 managed care reform laws; in 1997 alone, 90 such bills were introduced (Enthoven and Singer 1998, 96, 99).

If one assumes that policymakers do and should supply policies in response to stimuli grounded in "objective conditions," this rush to regulate managed care might be deplored as an inefficient obsession with making mountains of molehills. Focusing instead on risk—that nebulous connector of objective conditions with subjective anxieties—points out a different analytical path, one that in turn connects the construction of political stimuli with the content of policy responses. The analysis in this chapter tries to follow this path and discern those connections by the light of evidence drawn from interviews conducted in the second round of CTS site visits, in which researchers posed a range of questions about the origins, evolution, and results of managed care regulation to knowledgeable sources drawn from insurance plans (including MCOs), hospitals, physicians, advocacy groups, public officials, trade associations, and other groups. (For another cut at reading the evidence, see Ginsburg and Lesser 1999.)

Climate of Opinion

For most of the twentieth century, managed care was an exceedingly minor variation on dominant healthcare themes. This style of medical care delivery and financing became "news" in the early 1970s when the Nixon administration discovered the virtues of prepaid group practice, which it rechristened "health maintenance organizations," and sought new federal legislation to promote it. For two decades, slow progress kept managed care (as HMOs and their organizational hybrids came to be called) on the sidelines of health policy and public opinion (Brown 1983). By the mid-1990s, however, having registered huge enrollment gains, managed care had hit page one and prime time, and the message conveyed by the media was that, in the aftermath of the collapse of the Clinton plan for national health reform legislation, managed care had "taken over" the system de facto by default.

The "story," in essence, was this: Most of the population no longer "had" health insurance but instead "joined" health plans. Plan subscribers no longer chose physicians and hospitals freely but instead were limited to a closed panel selected by their plans. Physicians were no longer accountable solely to patients but also to plans and the purchasers who contracted with them. Patient care no longer reflected untrammeled professional judgment alone but also the insidious, and perhaps invidious, effects of administrative constraints and financial incentives that aimed to deter "inappropriate" care. Patients no longer simply enjoyed the protection of fringe benefits or public entitlements but also participated willy-nilly in a cost-containment exercise. Stated thus, managed care entailed controversial change on a broad scale and was major news indeed.

What consumers know of managed care in particular they learn from personal or family contacts with their health plans and from word of mouth; what they know of managed care in general they discover from the media. The evidence of personal experience and social communication stand in considerable tension, the character of which policymakers seek to gauge. Interviews in the 12 study sites plainly indicate that such personal satisfaction with managed care as consumers may personally enjoy is sharply and repeatedly challenged by "the news" about managed care reported in the press and on television, which, according to most respondents in most sites, is distinctively negative. (The main outliers in the study sample are Indianapolis, where one source described media coverage of managed care as "mildly positive," another found it "fair to neutral," and a third deemed it "negative"; and Seattle, where a highly activist and visible insurance commissioner seemed to draw publicity at the expense of coverage of managed care.)

Interviewees painted a fairly consistent picture of the organizational and professional forces that shape media coverage of managed care. News is what sells papers and attracts viewers; "horror stories" fill the bill admirably: "They like the drama of it all—reporting the fighting," said a consumer advocate in Boston; conversely, as a hospital official in Syracuse remarked, "good news is no story." Denials of care, especially of purportedly life-saving experimental procedures and transplants, and protracted legal battling are especially durable and eye-catching and encourage reporters to play their favorite "watchdoggy" role. A physician spokesman in Boston suggested that bad press goes with the territory: Ten years ago, big insurance companies took the heat; now the HMOs' turn has come. Be that as it may, defenders of MCOs complain that unfair coverage has become a standard operating procedure of the media (exceptions make news, denominators go unreported), that confidentiality rules hinder the ability of plans to correct errors by putting the facts in public view, that the media seem to view regulatory relief as a free lunch ("one finds no information in the Globe about costs," groused a business informant in Boston), and that coverage has turned a nation of plan members with no cause for alarm into confused legions of "worried well," crying out for costly protection against minuscule risks.

Nor does "local knowledge" about conscientious MCOs in quiescent communities suffice to restore balance to the public picture. In none of the 12 sites did respondents depict consumers seething with fury over the abuses of unscrupulous plans. On the contrary, the modal, indeed near-universal, image sketched reasonably contented consumers, responsible plans, and local media with few local problems to cover. Informants also remarked, however, that managed care bashing in the national media not only spurred consumers to doubt the evidence of their senses but also stirred local reporters to "scrounge," as a hospital administrator in Syracuse put it, for hometown hassles and horrors consistent with disquieting national news. Numerators, which a source in a Miami insurance plan called "terrible individual experiences" with managed care, fit well both the organizational agenda of media firms and the professional vocation of reportorial watchdogs. Denominators—the typical experience of populations—neither make news nor extenuate "abuses" by "powerful" interests.

The social construction of public opinion about managed care was well captured by a health plan executive in Miami who recounted a visit to him by a local reporter who had perused the files of official complaints against the plan, which, the reporter indignantly noted, ran to nearly 500 in the previous year. The plan executive remarked that his plan had more than a million-and-a-half patient contacts that year, to which the intrepid inquisitor rejoined that "even one complaint is too many." The public debate and reform agenda thus constructed is not about the performance of plans but about risk and not about the general merits and limits of managed care as a vehicle of health reform but about what impersonal formal organizations (MCOs) do, or could do, to consumers unwary or unlucky enough to fall under their wheels. The managed care "experience" thus constructed is quite literally Kafkaesque, and it is not odd that consumers should come to feel a diffuse desire for protection against errors and accidents supposedly waiting to happen. Nor is it odd that policymakers feel compelled to answer these demands by anticipating and addressing these risks (Rochefort 1998) or that providers labor to reap rewards from these political trends.

Capitalizing on the Climate

The widely publicized proposition that managed care threatens the health of the public has emboldened opponents and skeptics to promote laws and regulations that curb the managerial freedom of MCOs. Three groups are most active and influential in translating the public's inchoate yearnings for protection into public policies: physicians, advocates, and politicians.

1. *Physicians.* Physicians are the only group identified in all 12 study sites as prime movers for managed care regulation. This is entirely predictable: Organized medicine fought managed care tooth and nail for decades, has viewed its rising ascendancy with acute alarm, and now savors the chance to utter "I told you sos" as managed care comes into public disfavor. County and state medical societies across the 12 communities weigh in with proposals that would ease the economic plight of physicians confronting MCOs from within or without. These measures almost always include any-willing-provider laws, generally include mandatory POS options, and sometimes expand the legal liability of MCOs. Physician organizations also lend support to reforms that bear less immediately on their collective economic interests, such as the creation of "ombuds" positions, stronger grievance mechanisms and external appeal procedures, and consumer bills of rights and patient protection acts in general. In most sites, specialty groups add to this generic agenda of organized medicine their own vigorously pressed proposals that members of MCOs enjoy "direct access" to specialists either by appointing them as their primary care physicians or, more commonly, by gaining the right to schedule specialty appointments without prior referral by a PCP gatekeeper.

2. *Advocates.* A second, and seconding, source of demand for regulation of managed care is the "advocacy community"—a varied assortment of organizations that represent present or potential members of MCOs and fight to protect them from the threatening interests presumed to motivate the plans. Advocates include:

- organizations working to advance the needs of individuals suffering from chronic diseases such as cancer, lupus, multiple sclerosis, AIDS, asthma, substance abuse, mental illness, and other disabilities;
- organizations that enfold health issues in a broader agenda based on age or gender, such as AARP, Gray Panthers, Planned Parenthood, women's groups;
- organizations with a general mission to reform healthcare or protect consumers, such as Health Care for All in Boston, Universal Health Care Action Network in Cleveland, Citizens' Action in Northern New Jersey, Washington Citizen's Action in Seattle, Citizens Action and the Albany-based New York Public Interest Research Group in Syracuse; and
- economic or professional interest groups onto whose radar screen managed care has somehow come, such as nursing associations in Cleveland and Northern New Jersey; the United Auto Workers in Lansing; and lawyers with an eye on liability litigation who were mentioned by respondents in Miami, Northern New Jersey, and Phoenix.

The number of active advocacy groups and their influence on public policy differ substantially across the sites. In Greenville, Indianapolis, Lansing (excepting the powerful United Auto Workers), and Little Rock, such groups seem to be feeble and inconspicuous partly because in these sites managed care has not spread far enough to trigger much antipathy and advocacy and perhaps partly too because these "interests" are less numerous and less mobilized in these communities. In traditionally liberal Massachusetts and Boston, advocate groups are abundant and active: a source estimated that the coalition for reform of managed care in Massachusetts embraced 90 different organizations (not all of them advocacy groups to be sure). New York State is a hotbed of advocacy as well, and although much of it originates in New York City, it infuses state policies that in turn shape managed care in such sites as Syracuse. Citizens Action, a consumer group in New Jersey, was said to have 80 affiliated organizations, including several influential unions in this strong labor state. The other sites exhibit moderate levels of advocate activism, which fall between the relative quiescence of Greenville and the highly charged politics of Boston and Syracuse, or more accurately, of Massachusetts and New York.

The substantive agenda the advocate groups promote varies with the constituencies the groups represent. For example, organizations that speak for those with chronic conditions generally seek direct access to the specialists who presumably know best how to treat these conditions, and the natural political coalition between advocacy and specialist groups doubtless goes far to explaining why these measures tend to fare better politically than less broadly defended proposals such as any-willing-provider laws. Fuller disclosure of information on plan finances and practices, mandated coverage for clinical trials, creation or expansion of "ombuds" activities, and stronger members' rights to internal appeals and external review of contested treatment decisions find favor across the advocacy spectrum.

3. *Politicians.* The souring taste of press coverage and public opinion on managed care and the imploring by would-be public protectors in the advocate and physician sectors leave politicians little choice but to "respond" to demands for managed care regulation. How they respond, however, is by no means foreordained. On rare occasions, respondents mention officeholders who opine that managed care has slowed the growth of healthcare costs and that hasty regulation would be a mistake. Some politicians believe this but fear to say so in public. Many, probably most, wish the hullabaloo would pass but are ready to do as much or as little as necessary to protect their constituents and thus their political flanks.

Some political entrepreneurs legitimized the regulatory enterprise by taking the lead in promoting it, which of course generates further press coverage about the industry's failings and the candidate's correctives. Informants cited, for instance, Massachusetts's legislators who sought "mileage" from regulation, gubernatorial candidates in Arizona and Ohio who pushed patient-protection laws, and an assertive insurance commissioner in Washington. The political agenda usually starts with due-process-based measures that are simple to explain and hard, in principle, to oppose— more responsive grievance mechanisms, ombudsmen, information disclosure, fuller reviews and appeals, and mandatory POS. How much farther politicians go depends on the preferences and power of constituent groups that can do them good or ill. Direct-access laws draw strength from the above-noted specialist-advocate coalition. Where physician organizations are strong and opposition to them is weak, any-willing-provider laws, which are often assailed as a blatant assault on the very essence of man-aged care, may come to pass.

Alignment of interests among physicians, advocates, and politicians in augmenting regulation of managed care amid a climate of bad publicity and beleaguered public opinion is a powerful spur to action. Not surpris-ingly, many respondents see redoubled regulatory initiatives on the hori-zon. In Phoenix, "legislators are out to get us. There's strong feeling here," said a health plan administrator. In Syracuse, a respondent in the media expects that "more legislators will play doctor and pick a disease to pass legislation on." In Miami, explained an executive in a safety-net managed care plan, heavy negative media coverage of managed care "scares con-sumers and influences their opinions of managed care. Consequently, peo-ple want protection, choice, and quality, and the politicians see this and jump on the bandwagon." In Cleveland, a consumer advocate aptly sum-marized both the political logic of regulatory momentum and the indus-try's jaundiced view of it: [The politician's message to consumers is], "We are fighting the great fights. We will call you when it is over. The voice of the consumer is used, filtered, and amplified."

Countering the Case for Regulation

If physicians, advocates, and governmental critics of managed care were the whole political story, managed care would never have achieved its pres-ent prominence. This health-reform strategy came to center stage because it had powerful advocates of its own, notably purchasers who believed that managed care could solve their health-care cost problems and in the course of encouraging it nourished a sizable managed care industry with its own political muscle. Purchasers' continuing commitment to managed care and the presence of a powerful managed care lobby are formidable facts of political life that counter the appeals of regulation.

The growth of public, including of course employee, antagonism toward purchasers' handiwork has caused them some uncertainty and second thoughts: On the one hand, purchasers retain warm affection for the pros-pect that managed care will make healthcare more efficient, competitive, and businesslike; on the other hand, they know they lack conclusive in-sights into how MCOs work and cannot be sure that the public outcry and bad press are indeed much ado about nothing. Political prudence, there-fore, counsels that purchasers and plans repress inclinations to mount a vigorous positive public defense of managed care and concentrate instead on identifying and indicting the unanticipated consequences and costs of regulation.

The key opponents of managed care regulation in the 12 study sites are business associations (e.g., chambers of commerce, local purchaser coalitions, small business groups), sometimes aided by influential individual firms, and associations of MCOs, sometimes abetted by prominent individual plans. Antiregulatory activism, like the anti-managed care assaults to which it responds, tends to run higher in sites where managed care penetration is high or growing fast than it does in those where penetration is low or growing slowly from a small base. For example, respondents in Greenville noted the presence of a HMO lobby powerful enough to secure amendments to a law that had seemed to interfere with the ability of HMOs to establish POS plans, but they made no mention of organized business opposition to regulation. Neither managed care nor regulations to constrain it have many teeth in South Carolina. In Little Rock, Blue Cross Blue Shield and Prudential took up cudgels against a political push by organized medicine to enact an any-willing-provider law, but purchasers and plans are not disposed to dispute Arkansas's modest consumer-protection measures. Sources in Lansing and Syracuse remark both that their local workforces are highly unionized and that local MCOs refrain from managing care aggressively—a perceived correlation that invites causal conjectures. By contrast, Boston's 90-group coalition that works for regulation is challenged by a rich array of business groups—(e.g., the Boston Chamber of Commerce, Associated Industries of Massachusetts, the Massachusetts Health Care Purchaser Group, the Business Roundtable, and the Small Business Association) plus the Massachusetts Association of HMOs and the Harvard-Pilgrim Health Plan. Activism on one side does not invariably evoke its countervailing counterpart, however: The business community in New York State has been less assertive politically than the regulation-minded advocacy community, leaving much of the lobbying against regulation to the state's HMO conference.

Although the threat of regulation and the nature and extent of organized resistance to it vary across the communities, antiregulatory forces offer the same basic argument in all 12 study sites: Regulation will raise the costs of running MCOs, which will compel plans to raise their premiums and, in turn, will oblige employers to forego wage increases in order to pay for health coverage or to drop or curtail insurance coverage, thus increasing the number of uninsured. (Some brave souls occasionally add that consumer satisfaction with MCOs is high and that medical management can improve the quality of care, but these contentions evidently lack the clout of those based squarely on costs.) But a key link in the chain of antiregulatory argument—that incurring these costs to rectify errors and "abuses" is like using an elephant gun to shoot a fly—is generally left implicit or uttered sotto voce. Defenders of managed care thus generally start from the assumption that laissez faire is not a genuine option. The heated climate of public opinion and the broad constellation of groups that seek regulation assure that some regulation is a given; the opponents' goal is to render it as moderate and inoffensive as politically possible.

Purchasers and plans combine to stem the regulatory tide by means of three main stratagems. First, they try to portray for the public the bright side of managed care and the downside(s) of regulation. New Jersey's Association of Health Plans, for instance, held several press conferences to explain the industry's views on legislative proposals and consumer issues, but it found that the media were "not very interested." An interviewee in Phoenix explained that the state's HMO Association "tries to be proactive, to get out the message on the good things." This is a tricky business, however: Given the confidentiality of the medical details of particular cases, defenders of managed care can rarely refute definitively the dramatic insistence of critics that debate should rightfully focus on the tragedies of victims on whom MCOs have inflicted "terrible individual experiences." Assurances that the care in question was not so bad after all suggest a lack of commiseration, which hardly helps the industry's public image or relations.

Purchasers and plans know that their core arguments—in complex formal organizations mistakes do happen; the more accountable the system the more missteps will come to light; the costs of preventing errors should be reasonably calibrated to incidence and severity; in short, numerators should accompany denominators as reforms are contemplated—play best out of the public eye. Therefore, they lobby executive branch officials and legislators, seeking quietly to correct misunderstandings about the workings of managed care and to dramatize the costs of regulatory overkill, marshaling along the way data on the satisfaction of consumers, the plans' plans for quality improvement, and the additions to premiums that allegedly beset proposed rules.

Knowing that they cannot stop the regulatory juggernaut cold, antiregulatory forces generally fear that excessive obstinacy and obdurateness on their part could cost them political credibility and legitimize intrusive legislation. Consequently, in most study sites, purchasers and plans adopt a strategy of "working with" legislators, and often with physician and advocacy groups, and of "being at the table" in search of legislative compromises devoutly, albeit silently, sought by politicians who want to assuage public anxiety but do not wish to kill managed care and then be blamed for rising healthcare costs. In Massachusetts, an informant explained, legislators preferred to "work with plans" in order to avert heavy damage to managed care, which the Speaker of the House in that state credited with bringing health costs down. Indeed, one source contended that Harvard Pilgrim "wrote 90 percent" of a bill that had gone before the Massachusetts Senate. A respondent in Lansing noted that Michigan plans and purchasers "understood the potential for backlash" and worked to forestall it by "developing reasonable protections." Thus, the powerful Economic Alliance of Michigan—an organization of employers and unions—took the lead in reshaping a bill that physicians had introduced in the legislature. In Miami, an interlocutor observed that plans opposed regulation but negotiated with Florida's highly active Agency for Health Care Administration in hopes that reasonable regulation would head off aggressive legislation. In Arizona, "the plan association and the medical association have good relations and try to work together."

Anticipated Reactions

Education, lobbying, and negotiation are not the sole strategies by which MCOs, and the purchasers who defend them, work to counter the threat of regulation. As important as these "external" means (indeed probably more important) are internal changes in plan operations that aim to anticipate political reactions to the perceived shortcomings of managed care and thus, presumably, to cushion their impact. Surprisingly, these forestalling adaptations were not deplored in any study site as a threat to the survival or integrity of managed care or depicted as much more than minor nuisances. The most plausible explanation is that the problematic features of managed care that spur citizens to seek political redress also shape the decisions of those same citizen-consumers, and their employers, as they shop among competing plans. In anticipating regulatory reactions, then, plans may be simply and mainly doing what market signals simultaneously suggest. Heated pro and antiregulatory rhetoric may be more about means than ends. As a Boston respondent remarked, plans themselves are adopting much of what regulatory proposals would require, but they "just do not want to be dictated to by government." In Northern New Jersey, a source explained, MCOs in the state's Association of Health Plans joined in signing a prompt payment agreement and discussed strategies among themselves, and with physicians and drug companies, to enhance coverage for clinical trials, all in hopes of forestalling mandates.

Internal anticipatory strategies take several forms. First, because, as a Cleveland source noted, plans must "worry about the bad press they are getting," MCOs labor to persuade consumers that they are untainted by gag clauses, arbitrary termination of physician contracts for financial reasons alone, excessively short inpatient stays after childbirth, and drive-through mastectomies—practices that are highly publicized and highly offensive, albeit (say respondents) rare to nonexistent, even before all the critical hoopla.

Second, plans try to enhance the communication channels by which they learn what is on their members' minds. A Miami plan executive wondered: "All this talk of consumer protection? Why?" He then sketched his plan's effort to get to the bottom of things: "We work with an advertising agency. We invite calls to dialog with us on the issues. We got 10,000 calls, which gives us a rich database. We'll take what we heard and change the plan for the better." Sometimes unsettling information comes from outside. An informant in Syracuse recalled a survey, conducted by the local medical society, on how physicians perceived insurers; two plans scored poorly, made changes, and ranked higher the next time around. Many respondents emphasized that careful listening is a powerful management tool. Contending that poor customer service is the root of most discontent with managed care, a respondent from Syracuse argued: [many issues are] "management problems that lie outside the realm of regulation. Plans ought to have more consumer panels," such as (said he) those in Seattle's Group Health Cooperative of Puget Sound. As an interviewee in Cleveland put it: "We are all more sensitive than historically to consumer voices, and more sophisticated about getting the information—surveys, complaint analysis, ombudspersons, and so on." Third, therefore, enlightened plans try to correct misconceptions and gaps in consumer information by refining and expanding letters, advertisements, and other membership materials.

Fourth, plans modify the design of their products to honor intense consumer preferences, which, if neglected, might move members to switch plans, demand regulatory relief, or both. Because gatekeeping sits high on the average hit list, plans in most of the 12 communities permit members to go directly to at least some specialists, in hopes (often vain) of deterring direct access legislation that goes "too far." Such legislation in South Carolina had no impact in Greenville, contended a respondent who noted that his MCO already allowed such access. A Little Rock informant likewise characterized the consumer-protection laws in Arkansas as a minor concern for plans because protections were firmly in place—for instance, direct access to OB-GYNs and continuing coverage for 90 days with physicians who are dropped from a network. Interviewees in Miami and Phoenix cited direct access as an example of the new product plans proactively developed to keep and win customers. In general, the new look across the 12 sites highlights reduced gatekeeping, streamlined referrals, less-rigorous authorization procedures, and more extensive POS options, reforms in which politics and markets seem to reinforce each other's signals.

Fifth, because these motley efforts to keep members content can never be foolproof, plans and regulators race to improve mechanisms for the airing and resolution of complaints. Quicker grievance processes and easier resort to external appeals are the modal measures. Interviewees had no major objections to these steps, but two cautioned that they are not costless. One recalled that by commencing formal evaluations of informal complaints, an Indianapolis MCO had driven its official complaint rate higher. A Phoenix respondent portrayed readier resort to external appeals as a good news/bad news story: Appeals are few and most get resolved in favor of the plans, but the loss of even a few large ones means money damages and bad press to boot.

These several "reforms" obviously raise the cost of running MCOs above what they would be otherwise, and laying these impositions and extractions at government's door is an irresistible political weapon that antiregulatory forces brandish with predictable abandon. It is analytically impossible, however, to disentangle the sources and costs of managerial changes that result from the threat or introduction of public regulation from those originating in the calculations of a plan bent on keeping or expanding market share and preempting regulation by moving first. That regulation per se cannot now be proved or plausibly alleged to be highly onerous and costly does not mean that it will not become so, however. As a Boston source observed, plans expect to face tougher reporting requirements, higher administrative costs, and tighter operational restrictions. Presumably, this expectation will continue both to inspire anticipatory reactions within plans and to confound and confuse the causal connections between political and market sources of responsiveness to citizen-consumers.

Conclusion: Unreasonable Regulation?

On the surface, the politics of managed care regulation offer scant consolation to those (if any such remain) inclined to view public policy as an exercise in rational problem solving. If the newfound hegemony of managed care is a dangerous development that requires strict public supervision, the regulatory measures adopted by the states hardly seem equal to the job. If managed care is a good idea guilty of no more than minor miscues in practice, these same regulatory correctives amount to overhasty overkill. Reprising a familiar American political pattern, the regulatory process somehow ends up accused simultaneously of cowering before a powerful new industry and of disrupting promising market-building efforts. The "rational" response seems forever to lie beyond the political pale.

The evidence distilled here from the 12 study sites, however, encourages a closer look that challenges these pessimistic readings. One may well wish that denominators were more common and inflammatory numerators less so, but like it or not the issues driving regulation turn not on the assessment of the collective performance of managed care as a medical "style" but on the estimation and alleviation of individual risk. Americans may indeed pay unreasonably high prices to minimize small risks—from environmental pollution, say, or defective products, or contacts with health-care providers—but the myriad political expressions of that collective preference will not yield to stoic reminders that life is unfair and bad things can happen to good people. Culturally, anxieties over threats to health and safety from malfunctioning of the healthcare system itself ("first do no harm") may be especially, perhaps uniquely, intolerable. That "terrible individual experiences" are very rare is indeed no "excuse."

That errors happen(ed) as or more often in the unmanaged fee-for-service sector and that managed care, because it is more accountable than fee-for-service, risks looking worse by tracking its performance more closely and carefully are no extenuations either. Robert Frost was right: "something there is that doesn't love a wall." For better or worse, managed care manages care by erecting walls—limited provider panels, gatekeeping PCPs, authorization rules, financial incentives, and the rest—between consumers and the "unnecessary and inappropriate" medical care that providers would supposedly dish out wantonly otherwise. Purchasers and market-minded healthcare analysts welcome these walls as fortification against provider dominance and the costs it entails. Consumers distrust them and are skeptical of syllogisms proving that managed care providers will reliably hoist all care that is truly necessary and appropriate over such managerial obstacles as plans may deploy. Managed care regulation is largely about dismantling walls (for example, direct access laws that circumvent gatekeeping) or supplying ladders over them (for instance, more accessible grievance and appeals mechanisms). "Aggregate" costs and benefits (still less their ratio) are decidedly secondary considerations.

Managed care commenced as a minor movement sustained by physicians who viewed it, then called "prepaid group practice (PGP)," as a morally and professionally superior model of medicine (Brown 1983). After the federal government embraced PGP (a.k.a. HMOs) in 1970, this movement evolved uneasily into an industry dominated by for-profit firms and promoted by purchasers who viewed managed care as a means of curbing the autonomy of physicians and therewith slowing the rise of healthcare costs.

Once defended as a system of positive professional opportunities, managed care is now sold as a system of negative economic constraints. Purchasers and academic advocates have been far too quick to accept managed care as inevitable and indisputable progress in the healthcare field and as an offer consumers cannot, and should not, refuse either because they discern the impeccable logic of managed care or, more likely, because private and public purchasers leave them no real choice. As it happens, free choice of provider, physicians as advocates solely for patients' medical needs, and kindred quaint norms show substantial staying power; and the consumers (and physicians and advocates) inclined to defend them turn out to have a choice after all—namely, to demand public regulations that curb the managerial discretion of the managed care bureaucrats who seek to curb the autonomy of providers. The issues and stakes of the political struggle, in short, far transcend dry objective calculations of performance and risk under alternative forms of medical practice. The drive for regulation enjoys, moreover, deep political resonance rooted in American political tradition. As Moran (1999, 127) remarks, the rise of the managed care industry has created "precisely the kind of market structures, involving concentration in markets hitherto dominated by large numbers of independent entrepreneurs, which has historically triggered regulatory intervention in the American economy."

The policymakers who craft new rules in response to the demands of coalitions for regulation of managed care also, arguably, are less obtuse than casual or dogmatic impression suggests. In most states, the efforts of plans and purchasers to educate, lobby, and negotiate with political leaders who want to fine-tune managed care, not bury it, conduce to regulations that, respondents generally indicated, raise administrative costs marginally and perhaps a bit more, but are on the whole neither unmanageable nor unreasonable. The imagery of "command and control" regulation caricatures the politics of the process.

Equally important, many, perhaps most, policy responses to political demands parallel the plans' own organizational responses to preferences conveyed by the voice or exit of consumers, or their employers, shopping in competitive health plan markets. It is reasonable to assume both that the threat of regulation focuses plan attention on customer concerns, hastening efforts to address them, and that the plans' internal reactions that anticipate external intervention make regulators more willing to listen to, learn from, and find compromises with them. The political equilibrium that grows from the subtle interplay of regulatory demand and supply arguably achieves a higher rationality than tends to be recognized by the legions of participants and observers who dismiss the regulatory regimen as too little too late or too much too soon.

PART TWO

Community Reports

Local Organizations
Retain Market Dominance

In 1996, the Cleveland market appeared to be in turmoil. The community had experienced or was anticipating a number of high-profile mergers. Historic collaboration among providers had given way to competition, sparked by the market entry of two for-profit hospital systems. Local providers and plans, it seemed, were threatened. Yet, change in Cleveland did not materialize as expected. The proposed merger between Blue Cross and Blue Shield of Ohio and Columbia/HCA disintegrated. The three large local, not-for-profit institutions—the Cleveland Clinic, University Hospitals Health System (UHHS) and Medical Mutual of Ohio, the former Blue Cross and Blue Shield plan—remain dominant.

After an active period of deal making, focus now seems to have shifted to internal organizational issues. Key changes shaping the health system today include the following:

- Market concentration is increasing in the hospital sector.
- Hospitals are expanding high-end medical services.
- Plans are facing stiff price competition and internal administrative difficulties.
- Employers are not pursuing aggressive purchasing strategies.

Threat to Local Entities Subsides

Cleveland remains a community where leaders in business circles and local provider organizations are closely aligned through membership on the same community boards. These relationships are important forces shaping the direction of health system change in this market. Since HSC's

CLEVELAND DEMOGRAPHICS

	Cleveland, OH	Metropolitan areas above 200,000 population
Population, 1997 [1]	2,225,997	196,633,263
Population Change, 1990-1997 [1]	1%	6.7%
Median Income [2]	$27,967	$26,646
Persons Living in Poverty [2]	13%	15%
Persons Age 65 or Older [2]	15%	12%
Persons with No Health Insurance [2]	8.5%	14%

Sources: 1. U.S. Census, 1997; 2. Household Survey, Community Tracking Study, 1996-1997

1996 site visit, three local institutions—the Cleveland Clinic, UHHS and the former Blues plan, Medical Mutual of Ohio—have retained dominance in the market, while organizations without local roots have lost market position.

In the hospital sector, the market entry of two for-profit hospital chains—Columbia/HCA and Primary Health Systems (PHS)—prodded the two leading not-for-profit provider systems to increase their market share through acquisitions and affiliations. While competition in the hospital sector has intensified, several institutions continue to offer forums for collaboration, including Cleveland's hospital association and Cleveland Health Quality Choice (CHQC), a community-wide quality initiative.

The anticipated merger between Blue Cross and Blue Shield of Ohio and Columbia/HCA was expected to have a profound impact on the market. However, the proposed merger fell apart in March 1997, the same month that the national Blue Cross and Blue Shield Association stripped the insurance plan of its Blues trademark. The former Blues plan, renamed Medical Mutual of Ohio, reported a $95 million loss for 1996. But, since 1997, Medical Mutual has rallied successfully, maintaining its market share, key partnerships and its position as the dominant local plan.

To do so, Medical Mutual reportedly has pursued an aggressive pricing policy. In addition, the plan has made changes in key leadership positions, promoting staff and hiring back former employees. Medical Mutual also has maintained its close relationship with the Chamber of Commerce's small-business purchasing group and has successfully renegotiated its contract with the Cleveland Clinic. The plan's ability to retain its market position during the last two years appears to be further evidence of the importance of relationships and local identity in the Cleveland health care market. Its success was enhanced by the fact that Anthem, the Indianapolis-based plan that acquired the Blues trademark in the market, has not increased its share as anticipated.

Market Concentration Increasing

Both the Cleveland Clinic and University Hospitals have extended their reach throughout northeastern Ohio. They have developed additional primary and tertiary care capacity in partnership with their owned and affiliated providers. While both systems have grown, the Cleveland Clinic has clearly eclipsed its rival in market share. The Cleveland Clinic owns 40 percent of the hospital beds in Cuyahoga County and 30 percent in the broader six-county Primary Metropolitan Statistical Area (PMSA), compared with UHHS's 11 percent market share in Cuyahoga County and in the PMSA.

Since HSC's 1996 site visit, the Cleveland Clinic merged with the four-hospital Meridia Health System and the two-hospital Fairview Health System. It has also acquired Health Hill Hospital, a pediatric facility. At the same time, the Cleveland Clinic continues to build its Cleveland Health Network (CHN), which includes nine owned and 16 affiliated hospitals brought together under a super physician-hospital organization (PHO). To date, CHN has reportedly negotiated 40 contracts with 20 payers.

Most physicians who are not affiliated with one of the major hospital systems in the market remain in small groups. These physicians seem anxious about their futures and apprehensive about the increasing consolidation and influence of the hospital sector. Yet, there is little evidence of physician efforts to organize separately from hospitals. There are a few independent physician organizations, including multispecialty group practices, but none is seen as a major market force organizing physicians. Change may be on the horizon, however. At least two physician practice management companies have entered the market and may serve as potential future organizers for physicians.

While the two local not-for-profit hospital systems have grown, the two for-profit systems—Caritas, the partnership of Columbia/HCA and Sisters of Charity, and PHS—have suffered a loss of market position in the last two years. Initially, Columbia/HCA attempted to develop a statewide provider presence just as the Cleveland Clinic and UHHS were expanding their influence in the local market. More recently, Columbia/HCA has been preoccupied with its national crisis and the failure of its planned merger with Blue Cross and Blue Shield of Ohio. Meanwhile, PHS has been distracted by the financially troubled Mount Sinai Medical Center. Saddled with a large debt, the system has struggled to retain patients, while a number of its physicians have moved to UHHS and other hospitals.

Despite some concerns voiced in 1996, however, there are no reports that these for-profit systems have reduced their charity care. Both systems serve large numbers of low-income patients, and, in spite of their difficulties, apparently have continued to provide charity care for these patients at a relatively constant level. At the same time, MetroHealth, Cuyahoga County's public hospital, continues to be the leading provider of charity care and Medicaid services. The hospital maintains a close relationship with the Cleveland Clinic, participating as a lead member of CHN.

Mergers Spur Expansion of High-End Medical Services

Two years ago, Cleveland was viewed as a specialty-oriented health care market with considerable excess hospital capacity. This is even more true today. Providers continue their efforts to attract patients by increasing the availability of specialized services, with little observable effort to reduce costs and achieve efficiencies. Furthermore, the expiration of Ohio's certificate-of-need legislation has opened the door for new construction and technology investments by hospitals.

The Cleveland Clinic and UHHS are taking the lead in adding new services. The Cleveland Clinic is teaming up with Lake West Hospital to establish a heart clinic at Lake, and with Elyria Memorial Hospital for heart and urology services. According to some respondents, the Cleveland Clinic is also investing heavily in its pediatrics and oncology services, both long considered UHHS strengths. Meanwhile, UHHS is partnering with Southwest General Hospital to develop open heart surgery, pediatrics and cancer services, and with Lake Hospital for cancer services.

Providers, it seems, have felt little pressure to consolidate their services. Instead, hospital mergers appear to have propped up otherwise vulnerable hospitals and contributed to the expansion of highly specialized services. The major provider systems view their investments in tertiary care services at owned and partner hospitals as a way to establish loyalty and referral relationships. Some respondents, particularly those in outlying communities, are pleased that specialized services are now available locally. Other respondents question whether this trend is in Cleveland's best interest. They are concerned that expansion of highly specialized services may, over time, spread experience too thinly, diminish quality and increase costs.

To date, the Cleveland Clinic and UHHS have not done much to integrate services across their facilities, although both have consolidated some administrative functions. The two multihospital systems have achieved powerful market positions by increasing their size. But facility integration is a difficult and contentious process that is more complicated than negotiating a merger or acquisition and is often delayed by "stand still" agreements written into merger contracts. In the case of the Cleveland Clinic, integration efforts highlight cultural differences between salaried multispecialty group practice physicians at the Cleveland Clinic and independent, entrepreneurial staff physicians at newly acquired hospitals.

Plans Face Stiff Price Competition

There is clear price competition among health plans, driven in part by Medical Mutual's aggressive pricing to maintain market share. Premium levels have been flat or have declined during the past year. Purchasers reportedly are switching plans for lower prices less frequently because their current plans are willing to lower premiums to hang onto their business. Statewide, plans had small negative margins in 1997, according to the Ohio Association of Health Plans. In Cleveland, several plans, including Kaiser Permanente, reported losses for the year. Plans have reacted by changing executive leadership and shedding money-losing product lines, including Medicaid. Kaiser Permanente of Ohio removed its top Cleveland executives, merged its Cleveland and Akron operations and tried to raise premiums by 9 percent after posting a $36 million loss in 1997. Because of purchaser opposition, the actual premium increase was much lower. Kaiser continued to lose market share as employers turned away from traditional staff-model HMO products.

The relative stability of premiums may not be sustainable, and, in keeping with national trends, some predict an upturn for 1999. In Cleveland, health plans are trying to shift the focus of competition away from price to areas such as customer service and medical management. However, plans remain highly undifferentiated in the eyes of purchasers. Most plans share the same broad provider networks and are experiencing similar administrative problems.

For example, several respondents report that plans are having difficulty paying providers in a timely manner, in part due to implementation of new information systems. Others note that plans' patient information is often inaccurate, requiring providers to establish parallel information systems to manage patient care and insurance coverage.

Purchasers Seem Content with Status Quo

In contrast to some respondents' expectations, purchasers have not increased their demands for highly managed insurance products or turned to direct contracting to exert more control over cost and quality. Perhaps this is because purchasers are already getting what they want: low premium increases and very broad networks. In 1996, some observers thought that enrollment increases in Medicaid and Medicare managed care might stimulate an overall increase in managed care for the Cleveland market. Managed care penetration in both Medicaid and Medicare has indeed increased. Medicaid managed care enrollment in Cuyahoga County has risen from 54 percent to 88 percent of beneficiaries since 1996, while Medicare managed care penetration has increased from 8 percent to 21 percent. However, overall managed care penetration is only 27 percent. This rate is low compared with other markets and has not increased much, presumably because of the commercial sector's slow conversion to managed care.

Purchasers have not stepped up their efforts to pursue direct contracting, although the Health Action Council (HAC) of Ohio, a coalition of more than 90 corporate members representing about 325,000 covered lives, has moved forward with its planned Centers of Excellence initiative. The HAC negotiated global fees for 22 procedures and conditions with five hospitals. Based on data from CHQC and other sources, HAC preselected certain area hospitals to apply for a Center of Excellence designation.

Some community hospitals complained that this process was unfairly biased in favor of large academic hospitals. Five individual hospitals, including the Cleveland Clinic and University Hospital, eventually were selected for participation. So far, the initiative seems to have had little effect on local purchasing; only a handful of employers have signed on to purchase services through the program.

Medicaid Plans Face Low Rates and Declining Rolls

Ohio is moving ahead with mandatory managed care for most Medicaid enrollees in several parts of the state, including Cleveland. However, health plans report that it is increasingly difficult for them to break even, let alone make a profit, in the Medicaid market. Since 1996, Ohio has reduced its reimbursement rates for Medicaid managed care plans, while the number of plans has increased. Mirroring national trends, the numbers of Medicaid beneficiaries have fallen, probably reflecting the impact of welfare reform and a thriving economy.

Several Medicaid plans are having financial difficulties, and some, including United HealthCare, have recently withdrawn from the Medicaid market. Two of the remaining plans, both locally managed insurers serving mostly Medicaid eligibles, reportedly are faltering as well. According to the *Cleveland Plain Dealer,* the 35,000 Medicaid enrollees in one of these plans, Personal Physician Care, will be disenrolled by the state, apparently in anticipation of the plan's liquidation.

Respondents differed in their assessment of why Medicaid plans are having financial difficulties. Some cited the decline in the state's payment rates and increased competition among plans. Other observers believe that the rates are adequate and claim that inadequate management systems and poor infrastructure are to blame for plans' losses.

The number of Medicaid plans is expected to decline further as the state implements enrollment floors in each county. Under these new rules, only plans that enroll 10 percent or more of the eligible population will be allowed to contract with Medicaid. Disruption in health care services for Medicaid enrollees is not anticipated as a result of these changes. Most plans that contract with Medicaid to serve beneficiaries in Cleveland appear to include the same set of high-volume Medicaid providers in their networks.

Issues to Track

During the past two years, a small number of local institutions have increased their influence in the Cleveland market. The troubles of Columbia/ HCA and PHS, coupled with the failure of the proposed merger between Blue Cross and Blue Shield of Ohio and Columbia/HCA, created an opportunity for local not-for-profit systems to strengthen their market positions. They have moved aggressively to do so. As market developments continue to unfold, several key issues bear watching:

- Will local organizations continue to dominate the market?
- Will provider concentration ultimately increase service integration? Will concentration generate regulatory attention?
- How will specialty service expansions affect the market?
- Will health care premiums remain relatively stable? If not, how will purchasers react? How might plans differentiate themselves from one another?
- How will instability in the Medicaid market affect care for the poor?

Collaboration and Competition Coexist

The Syracuse health care market looks significantly different today from the way it did two years ago. Change, however, unfolded differently from how those in the market expected. At the time, there was concern that the powerful forces of change on the horizon would erode one of the hallmarks of Syracuse's health system—its collaborative character—but that remains intact. Changes causing concern in 1996 included the demise of hospital rate setting, mandatory Medicaid managed care, an emerging purchasing coalition and the entry of national managed companies into the local market. To date, none of these changes has had the impact anticipated because they either were delayed or did not yield the expected market response.

The following are the key changes that have taken place in Syracuse's health system since 1996:

- Newly formed physician groups are building market power.
- Two of the four leading hospitals are consolidating.
- Plans are pursuing regional partners.
- Preferred provider organizations (PPOs) and point-of-service (POS) plans are gaining enrollment.

Collaborative Structures Remain

The Syracuse health system continues to exhibit the strong collaborative spirit noted in 1996, with evidence of cooperative efforts across all sectors. The Hospital Executive Council (HEC), a long-standing group of hospital leaders, continues to pursue projects that benefit the four leading hospitals

Syracuse Demographics

	Syracuse, NY	Metropolitan areas above 200,000 population
Population, 1997[1]	740,771	
Population Change, 1990-1997[1]	-0.4%	6.7%
Median Income[2]	$24,855	$26,646
Persons Living in Poverty[2]	16%	15%
Persons Age 65 or Older[2]	14%	12%
Persons with No Health Insurance[2]	9.1%	14%

Sources: 1. U.S. Census, 1997; 2. Household Survey, Community Tracking Study, 1996-1997

or the community-at-large, where no single hospital has "staked out turf." Representatives of three health plans have recently formed a quality of care committee to develop guidelines and programs for asthma, diabetes and other chronic illnesses. In addition, the local health department has solidified a partnership with Medicaid HMOs to rationalize the provision of services between health plans and the public health sector and is working to extend the partnership to include commercial HMOs.

Despite these ongoing collaborative efforts, there is increased competition within the physician, hospital and plan sectors of the health system, and it is reportedly becoming more difficult for organizations to find common ground.

Physician-Owned IPAs Replace PHOs

A recent change in state regulation removed a barrier to the growth of independent practitioner associations (IPAs). IPAs are organizations of physicians that facilitate joint contracting with health plans without changing the ownership structure of the individual practice. Prior to 1996, an IPA in New York State could contract with only one managed care organization. Now, IPAs can contract with multiple organizations, offering a more flexible and powerful way for physicians to organize in the Syracuse market.

At the time of HSC's first site visit, most of the hospitals were developing physician-hospital organizations (PHOs) as a way to link physicians and hospitals. Today, IPAs have become the primary way of organizing physicians. While the PHOs were hospital driven, physicians are playing the leading role in the new IPAs. Roughly 90 percent of the physicians in Onondaga County belong to one of the four major IPAs.

These IPAs range in size from 300 to over 800 physicians. Each IPA has one hospital with which it is most closely affiliated, but these affiliations typically are not legally binding, raising the potential for physicians to shift alliances in much bigger blocks than they could before.

The IPAs are broad and overlapping. Physicians are in multiple IPAs, health plans contract with multiple IPAs and individual physician members still execute contracts with plans. IPA contracts stipulate that primary care physicians limit their participation to one IPA, but this has not been enforced. This practice has led to confusion over which contract applies to a particular patient. Most IPAs do not restrict membership or demand exclusivity for specialists, although several intend to limit membership for specialists in the future. It is a period of experimentation as physicians try to work out the best strategies to secure their market position.

Capitated payment arrangements were uncommon in Syracuse in 1996, but today physicians in IPAs are beginning to assume risk with the support of IPA structures. The typical arrangements allow physicians to assume risk at the IPA level, instead of having individual physicians take full financial responsibility for the care of enrollees who select them. Some contracts include primary care only, some involve all professional services and others involve shared risk for hospital care. Most individual physicians are still paid on a fee-for-service basis, and any risk is held at the IPA level. However, one IPA reportedly is capitating individual primary care physicians and subcapitating specialty care. Innovative for the Syracuse market, this arrangement is supported by a contract with a national physician management firm that provides the information infrastructure and experience to manage these contracts.

Because the health plan networks are typically broad and overlapping, they ostensibly give enrollees free choice of most physicians in town. The underlying physician arrangements, however, are increasingly keeping patients within more limited provider networks. Enrollee choice of primary care physician determines where they will be referred for specialty and hospital care. This differs by plan. Physicians Health Plan (PHP) enrollees currently choose among several subnetworks within the larger PHP network. In other health plans, physicians direct referrals to stay within their own subnetwork, which may be invisible to enrollees. Enrollees can still switch their primary care physician at will to access most providers, but the majority go where they have been referred.

IPA arrangements and associated health plan contracts have an impact on referrals beyond the relatively small number of covered lives involved.

For example, a primary care group has contracted with selected specialists to handle referrals for a capitated rate. These specialists are likely to get all that group's referrals, not just those covered by the capitation contract, leading to fewer referrals to other specialists. So far, the IPAs have not attempted to influence physician care delivery patterns to reduce cost or improve quality.

There is no consensus about whether IPAs have increased the power of physicians in the market, increased competition among physicians and/or diminished the historical market prominence of the hospitals. Physicians are clearly becoming more proactive in the market, but the ultimate impact of their efforts remains to be seen.

Consolidation Leaves Three Hospital Systems

An affiliation between two of the four leading hospitals in the Syracuse area is underway. In 1996, respondents predicted hospital consolidation, but varied in their assessment of which entities would be involved. The way in which consolidation actually unfolded is as much a result of collaboration as competition.

Two local studies were undertaken to project the future need for hospital capacity in Syracuse, and both projected significant overcapacity in the near future. Bilateral talks about mergers and affiliations took place among various pairs of hospitals. The result was a plan to bring Community General Hospital and Crouse Health together as separate corporations in a single holding company. The two hospitals expect the arrangement to combine complementary geographic service areas, create economies of scale and improve their contracting position with health plans. Although the other hospitals in Syracuse reportedly do not perceive this affiliation as an immediate threat, one health plan respondent noted that with Crouse's recent operational improvements, low cost-position and savvy leadership, the new organization could be well positioned to seek volume at the expense of its competitors. Together, Crouse and Community General were responsible for just over half of the admissions to Syracuse hospitals in 1997.

Upsurge in Premiums, Plans Seek New Markets Regionally

After several years of aggressive competition and flat premiums, managed care plans in Syracuse are struggling to recoup operating losses. Opinions differ about who started the price war and whether the intent was to capture market share from managed care competitors or from traditional plans. Regardless, the result was an increased differential between HMO and indemnity plans, and HMO penetration increased. Despite reported enrollment gains, a number of health plans posted substantial financial losses last year and raised rates in 1998 by 9 to 16 percent. Health plans project further increases for 1999.

Several developments spurred by the price war have changed what had been a landscape dominated by strong local players.

- The position of PHP, the historically dominant local HMO started by four Syracuse hospitals, was weakened due to underwriting losses fueled by the price war, lower returns on a large contract than expected and the distraction of management by its merger discussions. PHP's recently announced merger with Health Care Plan of Buffalo may dilute the local character of PHP, but becoming a regional player may also help it survive.
- Blue Cross and Blue Shield of Central New York (BCBSCNY), which covers the Syracuse area, recently merged with the Rochester and Utica-Watertown Blues plans. The new organization is pricing its managed care products more competitively and lowering payment rates to physicians.
- Several national health plans have entered the Syracuse market by acquiring plans with a local presence, including CIGNA, United HealthCare, Kaiser Permanente and Aetna/U.S. Healthcare. To date, however, the growth of national health plans in Syracuse has been held back by internal issues related to mergers and lack of effective local marketing strategies.

The period of flat to declining premiums following the 1996 site visit may partly explain why purchaser activity did not progress as expected. At that time, the Purchasing Coalition of Central New York was attracting considerable attention. Some viewed the emergence of this group as a sign that businesses were attempting to drive down costs. In late 1996, the coalition granted PHP an exclusive contract for administrative services only. Since then, some of the original coalition members dropped out. While a few new ones have been recruited, the PHP contract covers only 20,000 lives, well short of the coalition's goal of 50,000.

Purchasers, however, are beginning to react to the recent premium increases. One large national employer offered to meet with local providers to help one plan bring down its costs. This is an unusual move in a market populated by branch offices of national firms that have not typically played a role in local health care dynamics.

The recent rate increases are eroding the differential that had developed between the cost of traditional benefit plans and HMOs. Consequently, employers—many of whom pass premium changes along to their employ-ees—are reportedly experiencing an enrollment trend away from managed care benefit offerings.

At the same time, the high single- to double-digit premium increases have led plans to introduce tighter network products so that employers can avoid some of the cost increases associated with current broad network products. So far, these tighter network products have been popular only with smaller, more cost-conscious employers. But plans expect more em-ployers to offer these products in 1999 and more employees to switch if they face increased cost sharing.

Despite all the activity among managed care plans and the focus of the provider community on positioning for managed care, the majority of the population in Syracuse is still covered under non-HMO health insurance plans. Current managed care penetration is estimated to be 19 percent, compared with 14 percent in 1996.

Cautious Response to Deregulation

In 1996, it was expected that deregulation of hospital rates would in-crease competition among hospitals in the Syracuse market, lower hospi-tal rates and put graduate medical education programs in jeopardy. Since deregulation's implementation in 1997, however, its actual effect has been more moderate. Both hospitals and health plans were largely un-prepared for the rate negotiation process in terms of information infra-structure and management experience. Syracuse hospitals took steps to reduce costs in anticipation of the need to offer more competitive rates, but did not move to undercut their competitors in the first two cycles of negotiations since rate setting ended. The health plans appear to have limited leverage in negotiations because of the small number of hospi-tals in Syracuse, their different mix of services and market demand for choice.

There are differing opinions about how hospitals and health plans in Syracuse fared under deregulation. Health plans claim they are paying more for hospital services today than under rate regulation, and hospitals claim they are getting less. Rural hospitals—usually the only players in a community—have more leverage and reportedly negotiated more favorable rates. Overall, hospitals are doing better financially than they were in 1996, while many of the health plans have incurred substantial losses. However, these trends are similar to what is happening on the national level for hos-pitals and plans, so deregulation may not be the primary driver with re-spect to financial position.

Medicaid Managed Care Delayed

In 1996, it was expected that Medicaid managed care would be a key driver of the market move toward managed care, but this has not been borne out. Voluntary enrollment in Medicaid managed care, in place in some form since 1988, has declined over the past two years. New York State received federal approval to implement mandatory Medicaid managed care in 1997, but delayed statewide implementation due to administrative complexities. The state is focusing its efforts on New York City and is proceeding county by county. Implementation in Onondaga County, where Syracuse is located, is awaiting results of a recent Health Care Financing Administration site visit.

Overall, Medicaid managed care enrollment has declined in Syracuse since 1996. Since that time, the state reduced its Medicaid payment rates. A number of health plans serving Syracuse's Medicaid population dropped out because of the rate decreases and the restrictions on marketing practices that made it difficult and costly to attract enrollees. The state then increased rates, but has not attracted reentrants or new Medicaid plans to Syracuse. The health plan sponsored by the local community health center expanded its provider network, but did not absorb all the displaced enrollees.

Although Medicaid managed care has been limited in Syracuse, it may have had a positive impact on access to primary care for the Medicaid population. The local health department reports less demand for preventive health services, which it attributes to better access to care through Medicaid managed care plans. Fears that Medicaid managed care would result in a shift in volume away from the area community health center and harm its ability to care for the uninsured poor have not materialized, largely because much of the Medicaid managed care enrollment is in Total Care, the health plan sponsored by the community health center. Other health plans are not actively competing for enrollment at this time.

Consumers Get Patient Protection Laws, More Choice in Plans

At the same time that it has been deregulating the hospital sector, New York State has enacted one of the most comprehensive managed care consumer protection laws in the country. These laws address information disclosure, external and internal appeals and grievance procedures, gag clauses, due process protections, procedures to determine medical necessity, 48-hour stays for deliveries and mastectomies, chiropractic care, direct access to specialists and prompt settlement of health care claims.

There is widespread perception that there has been little public demand locally for these regulations. As one respondent put it, "Syracuse plans were not engaging in the restrictive practices addressed by this legislation." With the exception of the chiropractic mandate, respondents indicated that these regulations have not had a dramatic effect on plan policies, procedures or costs other than increasing the administrative burden on health plans.

While legislative changes reportedly have had little impact on health plan structure, they have helped to foster growth of less restrictive products. One direct by-product of hospital rate deregulation is the emergence of PPO products. Under New York State's previous rate regulation system, only licensed HMOs could negotiate rates with hospitals, so there was no incentive to form PPOs. Now that this restriction has been eliminated, national carriers are introducing PPO products, which are beginning to build an enrollment base in Syracuse.

POS products are also becoming more popular despite the fact that most health plans contract with all of the hospitals and most of the physicians. United HealthCare has introduced an open access product with no gatekeepers, and Blue Cross and Blue Shield offers a triple-option product in which enrollees can choose among varying levels of benefits and broader or more narrow networks at the point of service.

The new options appeal to employers and consumers who value provider choice and easier access to specialty care. However, expected premium increases may again push the market toward the more restrictive managed care products.

In addition, many plans have introduced new administrative-services-only products to serve the increasing number of employers who self-insure. There are differing opinions as to whether the new legislation, coupled with other regulations, including community rating, is driving employers to self-insure.

Issues to Track

Although change has not unfolded as predicted, the Syracuse market looks significantly different from how it did two years ago. New organizations have emerged, the balance of power is shifting and referral patterns are becoming more distinct. As HSC documents change in communities across the United States, key trends to track in Syracuse include the following:

- What impact will physician organizations have on the Syracuse market?

- Will competition overtake the collaborative nature of the health care community?
- What will be the impact of deregulation—and new regulation—on the market?
- How will purchasers respond to premium increases: Will more restrictive forms of managed care take hold?
- How will all these changes affect residents in Syracuse?

Market Stabilizes around Five Large Organizations

After a series of health plan and hospital mergers leading up to HSC's site visit in 1996, Boston's health care market entered a period of greater organizational stability. This trend continues today. Five nationally renowned not-for-profit organizations still dominate—two large care systems based in academic medical centers, Partners and CareGroup, and three large health plans, Harvard Pilgrim Health Care, Tufts Associated Health Plan and Blue Cross and Blue Shield of Massachusetts (BCBSM). While there have been some shifts in the competitive position of these entities, no single organization or sector controls the market.

Alongside this continuity there have been important changes in the market:

- Health plans have assumed a defensive posture as they encounter increased anti-managed care sentiment.
- The focus of large care systems has shifted from finding partners to managing large networks and risk contracts.
- Medicaid enrollment has increased, but consolidation, market exits and state contracting changes have left fewer plans serving this population.

Boston Retains Distinctive Market Features

The Boston health care market—with a 46 percent HMO penetration rate—has several features that make it different from other high managed care communities. It is dominated by three well-regarded not-for-profit health plans and is influenced by an activist government with a strong

BOSTON DEMOGRAPHICS

	Boston, MA	Metropolitan areas above 200,000 population
Population, 1997[1]	4,369,071	
Population Change, 1990-1997[1]	1.8%	6.7%
Median Income[2]	$29,996	$26,646
Persons Living in Poverty[2]	10%	15%
Persons Age 65 or Older[2]	14%	12%
Persons with No Health Insurance[2]	9.1%	14%

Sources: 1. U.S. Census, 1997; 2. Household Survey, Community Tracking Study, 1996-1997

consumer orientation. A large proportion of families report being satisfied with their health care—more than in other HSC study sites with high managed care penetration. There are more hospital beds and physicians per capita, and health costs are significantly higher than the national average. These costs are viewed by purchasers, plans and providers as a reasonable trade-off for access to Boston's academic medical centers, key contributors to the local economy. Indeed, desire to maintain teaching and research capabilities was the main justification for the merger of Massachusetts General Hospital and Brigham and Women's Hospital that created Partners in 1993.

While cost cutting has not been the major focus of attention, some organizations have tried to reduce operating costs in the last two years. BCBSM reports that it eliminated 50 percent of its staff in an effort to shed unprofitable business and streamline its operations. Boston Medical Center also made significant cuts, and Harvard Pilgrim recently announced plans to lay off at least 100 staff members.

At the same time, employers are accepting moderate increases on an already high premium base, although they are pushing plans to deliver added benefits and better customer service in return. Premiums in Boston rose by about 3 to 5 percent in 1998, on par with the national increase of 3.3 percent. Many observers predict that plans will press for larger premium increases in the range of 8 to 10 percent for 1999 because of their poor financial performance over the last two years.

Government Continues to Act as a Shaping Force

State government has long played a major role in shaping the Boston health care market. Extensive protections and mandates are already in place in Massachusetts, and the state government continues to play an active, behind-the-scenes role in shaping the health care market. Health care organizations pay close attention to concerns voiced by legislators and government officials and often proactively change their strategies to address these issues. At the same time, health care organizations try to achieve their competitive goals through policy initiatives.

Although little new legislation has been passed over the last two years, much debate has taken place on managed care issues. Reforms that were proposed in 1998 but did not pass would have introduced more state oversight of managed care plans, instituted a standardized appeals process and increased state-mandated services by requiring coverage for reasonable emergency room visits. Similar laws are expected to be proposed in the next legislative session.

As in the past, this year's managed care proposals mobilized employers and health plans in opposition. The managed care debate also brought physicians and consumer groups into an unprecedented alliance in support of increased state oversight. The recent legislative effort has had a lasting impact on the market. Plan respondents indicate that local HMOs that have long been highly regarded have suddenly become unpopular.

As Plans Retrench, Provider Systems Strengthen Market Position

Confronted by increasing anti-managed care sentiment, plans are perceived to be assuming a lower profile than two years ago. They seem to have limited their scope of activities, selling off owned provider capacity, reducing product lines and transferring some responsibilities to providers. BCBSM sold its nine health clinics to MedPartners to support its goals of generating cash and returning to core functions. Harvard Pilgrim spun off its 14 health centers, the centerpiece of the original Harvard Community Health Plan, into a physician-directed enterprise, Harvard Vanguard.

The major plans have pursued regional strategies by affiliating with, buying or establishing plans in the other New England states to offer products to multistate employers. At the same time, there have been shifts in the market position of the three large plans. Harvard Pilgrim is still the largest plan in Massachusetts, but Tufts has moved into second place, due in large part to the strength of its Secure Horizons Medicare managed care product. BCBSM, once the largest insurer by far, is now in third place. While the Blues plan appears to be on the upswing, it has faced significant problems over the last few years, with financial losses that prompted close oversight by the state's Department of Insurance and an enrollment freeze on its Medicare risk plan initiated by the federal Health Care Financing Administration.

Meanwhile, local provider systems appear to be operating from a position of relative strength, as they move from a period of finding partners to one of making existing partnerships work. They have expanded their range of activities in the last two years, as they implemented mergers, built networks and established risk management infrastructures. Respondents point out that large academic hospitals were notably silent during recent managed care debates in the legislature. These organizations seem well served by having plans take the heat from consumers and advocates.

Other health care entities in Boston are trying to increase their market power, by affiliating either with the five major organizations or with other entities. For example, Neighborhood Health Plan (NHP), a Medicaid HMO formed by the city's community health centers, was recently acquired by Harvard Pilgrim Health Care. New England Medical Center, one of the last unaffiliated academic medical centers, was recently acquired by Rhode Island-based Lifespan. And Lahey Clinic recently announced a new partnership with CareGroup, after Lahey's merger with the New Hampshire-based Hitchcock Medical Center fell apart. These changes highlight the continued importance for plans and providers of being part of large, regionally powerful organizations.

No Immediate Gain Seen from Hospital Consolidation

By the time of the 1996 site visit, three large care systems had formed from a series of mergers with the stated goals of gaining market power and reducing excess capacity. Different consolidation strategies were pursued, with some integrating more than others. Two years later, it appears that the systems that did more to integrate and consolidate have not yet seen a payoff in market position.

- Partners retained the autonomy of its two flagship hospitals, Massachusetts General and Brigham and Women's, and sought integration opportunities that promised immediate returns and little opposition, especially from influential department chairs. While most of the managed care contracting and many administrative functions such as human resources and purchasing were centralized, Partners' two main hospitals have remained operationally and clinically autonomous. The degree of independence of the hospitals was demonstrated when Massachusetts General opened an obstetrics unit, even though Brigham and Women's is the pre-eminent maternity hospital in the area. Although a significant downsizing in Boston's academic hospital capacity has long been predicted, Partners' two academic institutions have opened previously closed beds during the past two years to accommodate increasing patient volume.

- CareGroup devoted extensive effort and resources to combining Beth Israel Hospital and Deaconess Hospital into one entity. Significant progress has been made, including merging all departments and appointing single department chiefs. However, the process has been contentious and difficult. According to several reports, most of the chiefs selected for the merged departments were from Beth Israel, alienating many Deaconess physicians. While CareGroup reports that it has been successful in reducing costs as a result of the consolidation, some respondents note that its internal focus in the last two years has damaged the system's competitive position. However, the recently announced partnership with Lahey Clinic may improve CareGroup's standing in the market.

- The Boston Medical Center merger consolidated Boston City Hospital (BCH) and Boston University Medical Center (BUMC) into one entity. Benefits of the merger include complementary clinical expertise and substantial cost savings. However, Boston Medical Center is viewed by many as being financially and operationally vulnerable. The consolidation also brought out cultural conflicts. Boston City's physicians tended to be primary care-oriented, while BUMC's physicians were more academic and subspecialty-focused. Physicians from BCH were concerned that the BUMC doctors would not support the public hospital's mission of community service and care for the poor. These concerns, however, appear to have subsided somewhat since the merger was implemented.

Overall, Partners appears to be in a better competitive position than the other two large care systems, CareGroup and Boston Medical Center, which both did more to integrate and consolidate. However, some have noted that Partners' success may hinge more on the reputation and access to capital of its two hospitals than on its integration strategy.

Large Care Systems Focus on Managing Risk Contracts

The number of lives covered under providers' risk-based contracts has increased substantially over the last two years, and the two large academic medical center-based systems—Partners and CareGroup—have turned greater attention to implementing these contracts and managing their provider networks. Although these agreements still represent a relatively small share of the academic hospitals' business and reportedly have not been profitable, they are seen to be important because the number of risk contracts is expected to grow, and because the networks are significant referral sources for the hospitals. The two systems have apparently invested heavily in the information and staff infrastructure needed to support these contracts, and observers predict they will push for payment increases when their plan contracts are renegotiated.

Partners and CareGroup have established management service organization (MSO)-like structures to manage this business, and these entities are now considered the dominant physician contracting organizations in the Boston market. Partners Community HealthCare, Inc., has 915 primary care physicians in its network, while CareGroup's Provider Services Network has about 500. Both organizations have reportedly slowed acquisitions of physician practices, favoring affiliations and joint ventures.

For most of these risk contracts, the MSO is slated to receive 70 to 80 percent of the premium for enrollees from plans. Population-based budgets are established, and providers are paid on a fee-for-service basis with year-end reconciliation. The large care systems pass some of the risk along to risk units, each consisting of a group of physicians, such as the Massachusetts General physician group, and its affiliated hospital. Risk is assigned to these units based on the enrollee's choice of primary care physician.

The increasing focus on risk contracts has highlighted the underlying tensions between academic medical centers and community hospitals about how to structure payments to the multiple risk units within their networks. Physicians affiliated with the academic medical centers want to institute risk adjustment methodologies to avoid penalties for attracting sicker patients who require more services.

Meanwhile, physicians based at community hospitals are concerned that the drive for better risk adjustment methodologies is part of a larger academic medical center strategy to attract patients who had historically received care at community hospitals. This concern may ultimately drive community hospitals and their physicians to seek contracting vehicles that are less closely tied to the academic medical centers.

Concerns Raised about Control of Referrals and Care Management

With the increase in risk contracts comes the critical issue of who controls referrals. Partners and CareGroup are directing patient referrals for at-risk business to their own affiliated physicians and hospitals. This raises concerns among health plans that patients will not have full access to the broad networks they are building and promoting in response to purchaser and consumer demands.

Plan reactions to provider referral management have varied. Harvard Pilgrim Health Care allows primary care providers who are at risk to make their own referral decisions but also allows enrollees to switch primary care providers at any time. Tufts Associated Health Plan has told providers who accept risk that enrollees must have access to the full Tufts network. BCBSM is also concerned about referral restrictions, especially since its signature asset is the breadth of its network, but it has not taken any action to counter referral management by providers, in part because it believes that could generate negative publicity.

The large care systems also want to control more care management functions to obtain a larger share of the capitated dollar. So far, plans have retained many care management responsibilities, including functions such as tracking and developing care plans for enrollees with chronic diseases. Plans have resisted handing over more responsibility on the grounds that care systems have not demonstrated their ability to implement system-wide quality improvement initiatives.

Medicaid Enrollment Increases, but Fewer Plans Participate

Medicaid enrollment increased significantly as a result of program expansions in 1997 and 1998, when more than 100,000 children and adults gained coverage under the state's Medicaid program, MassHealth. With these expansions in place, some speculate that the state may reduce funding for the uncompensated care pool, which pays for health services for eligible uninsured.

The largest recipients of uncompensated care pool dollars, Boston Medical Center and Cambridge Hospital, have developed their own managed care programs to attract MassHealth enrollees and the uninsured. These two hospital systems negotiated higher Medicaid payments and approval to develop shadow managed care programs for the uninsured. Under these new programs, the hospitals use pool dollars to fund a comprehensive package of services for the uninsured. Rather than receiving treatment on an episodic basis, the uninsured enrollees will be linked with primary care providers and have access to preventive services.

While the number of Medicaid eligibles has grown, the number of HMOs serving the Medicaid market has declined. Two commercial plans in the market—BCBSM and Tufts Associated Health Plan—are no longer contracting with the state's Medicaid program. The two plans had a combined enrollment of more than 60,000 Medicaid recipients and very broad provider networks. BCBSM withdrew because it was losing money on Medicaid. Tufts, which was also reported to have lost money on Medicaid, indicated it could not comply with the state's increased reporting requirement along with the information technology demands presented by year 2000 computer problems.

With these two plans out, Harvard Pilgrim is the only remaining commercial plan serving the Boston Medicaid market. At the same time, the plan has stopped enrolling Medicaid beneficiaries in its large Pilgrim network, relying instead on the narrower networks of Harvard Vanguard and NHP providers. While beneficiaries still have access to a very broad network of providers under the state's primary care case management (PCCM) program it maintains as an alternative to HMOs, there are concerns about the implications of these changes. According to market observers, changes in plans' participation in Medicaid indicate that HMOs with broad and more loosely managed networks have had trouble surviving with the current rates. The state's response to these new challenges remains to be seen.

Issues to Track

In the past two years, the large academic care systems have grown stronger, and tensions have increased between these organizations and the three leading health plans. At the same time, Boston's health care system has retained many of its unique attributes: high managed care penetration, high costs, renowned plans and academic hospitals and an activist government. Emerging issues that could upset this stability include the following:

- How will large care systems like Partners and CareGroup handle risk adjustment and referrals internally? What will be the effect on academic medical centers' relationships with community hospitals?
- Will health plans cede more plan responsibilities, including care management, to providers?
- Will Medicaid change its purchasing strategy in light of health plan consolidation and exits from the Medicaid market?
- What impact will managed care legislation have on the market, whether enacted or just anticipated? Do these recent legislative proposals signal an emerging shift in Boston residents' longstanding favorable view of managed care?

Capacity Expands in Unrestrained Market

In 1996, Little Rock was still a largely traditional health care market, with a surplus of facilities and services, limited health maintenance organization (HMO) enrollment and predominately fee-for-service arrangements. However, several developments-including entry of national health care firms, the creation of a state purchasing pool and new alliances between major hospitals and health plans—signaled the promise of significant change. Yet by 1998, these changes had not unfolded as expected. National firms have not usurped locals' market share, and fee-for-service continues to prevail. With few outside pressures, the alliance between the dominant insurer, Arkansas Blue Cross Blue Shield, and the largest hospital system, Baptist Health System, remains a focal point of competition.

Among the key changes shaping Little Rock's health care system today:

- Local providers and plans are partnering with other national firms to bolster their market position and hold the large insurer-hospital alliance in check.
- Physicians are establishing numerous ambulatory surgery centers and merging their practices in an attempt to protect their income and clinical autonomy.
- Both inpatient and outpatient capacity continue to expand, despite existing excess.

Market Shaped by Few Restraints

The Little Rock health care market continues to have few restraints imposed by purchasers or state policy. In an economy dominated by small

LITTLE ROCK DEMOGRAPHICS

	Little Rock, AR	Metropolitan areas above 200,000 population
Population, 1997[1]	552,194	
Population Change, 1990-1997[1]	7.4%	6.7%
Median Income[2]	$24,447	$26,646
Persons Living in Poverty[2]	14%	15%
Persons Age 65 or Older[2]	12%	12%
Persons with No Health Insurance[2]	16%	14%

Sources: 1. U.S. Census, 1997; 2. Household Survey, Community Tracking Study, 1996-1997

firms, there has been little organized purchaser activity, although private purchasers' sensitivity to both premium increases and restrictions on provider choice has driven competition. The only significant purchaser initiative in recent years was the creation of the Arkansas State Employee/Public School Personnel Insurance Board in 1995. This initiative merged state employees and public school personnel under a joint procurement process now covering about 73,000 individuals statewide, most of whom live in the Little Rock area. The new purchasing process, along with a requirement that employees pay a greater share of the premium for more expensive plans, spurred rapid growth in managed care and prompted plans to position themselves to compete for enrollment.

Aside from this purchasing initiative, however, the state continues to play a limited role in shaping Little Rock's health care market. Arkansas repealed its certificate-of-need regulations for acute care services soon after the federal mandate for these regulations was lifted, and state legislators rejected health reforms proposed in 1995, reinforcing their preference for a health system driven by market forces rather than one shaped by government. Ironically, at the same time, legislators passed a far-reaching any willing provider law that would have required all plans—including those protected by the Employee Retirement Income Security Act (ERISA)—to contract with all providers willing to accept the plan's fee schedule and other terms and conditions. However, the courts struck down the law, first in 1997 and again on appeal in 1998—thereby preventing it from being enforced.

Unlike the vast majority of states, Arkansas has not moved to enroll the Medicaid population in HMOs, relying instead on a primary care case management (PCCM) program as the major initiative to improve access and control costs for this population. The only other new policy development over the past two years has been the implementation of the state's children's health insurance program, separate from the federal Children's Health Insurance Program. The state's program has extended coverage to approximately 36,000 children—one-third of projected total enrollment—since it began in September 1997. While the program is expected to help begin to alleviate the state's high rate of uninsurance, which is disproportionately concentrated among children and young adults, it is unlikely to have a major impact on the shape of competition in the market.

Threat of Outside Entrants Fades

At the time of HSC's first site visit in late 1996, it was anticipated that the entry of outsiders would change Little Rock's health care environment. For the past several years, a number of national health care companies had come to Little Rock seeking to build market share. Among the most significant changes in the market was the growing presence of Columbia/HCA. Columbia entered the market in 1994 as a result of its national merger with HCA. The newly merged entity assumed control of HCA's local hospital, Doctors Hospital, and shortly afterward, purchased the largest medical group in Little Rock. Then, in early 1997, Columbia/HCA announced plans to acquire Southwest Hospital and increase its market share through additional acquisitions, sparking concern among local providers about the company's growing role in the market. At the same time, national plans such as United HealthCare, Prudential HealthCare and Healthsource, Inc., were mounting a competitive challenge to local health plans. The entry of these national plans intensified premium competition and plans' marketing campaigns.

During the past two years, the anticipated threat of outside entrants failed to materialize, as national firms did not capture significant market share from locally based competitors. Many of these firms now have either reduced their presence or retreated from the market altogether. After it failed to garner its anticipated market share and against a backdrop of national Medicare fraud allegations, Columbia/HCA quickly exited the Little Rock market. Both Prudential HealthCare and CIGNA, which purchased Healthsource, appear to be backing away from Little Rock, although they continue to offer products locally, particularly to service their national accounts. These plans reportedly have not been successful in leveraging the oversupply of hospital beds and long lengths of stay needed to generate anticipated profit margins. While respondents note that United HealthCare appears to have remained a viable national plan in the Little Rock area, it is clear that, despite outside pressures, Arkansas Blue Cross Blue Shield has retained its dominant position in the market.

Local Entities Team Up with Other National Firms

Meanwhile, local providers and plans have established affiliations and joint ventures with other national organizations that have bolstered their market positions. The Arkansas Heart Hospital, a joint venture between local cardiologists and the national cardiac care management company MedCath, Inc., continues to build presence in the market. Discontent with local hospitals reportedly spurred two groups of cardiologists to approach MedCath and establish The Arkansas Heart Hospital, which opened in early 1997. Since then, the hospital has lured an estimated 10 to 20 percent of cardiac surgical volume away from the two major Little Rock hospital systems. Market observers speculate that the hospital's market power ultimately will depend on its ability to secure managed care contracts. To date, however, most of the hospital's volume has come from Medicare fee-for-service patients.

In late 1997, St. Vincent Health System, one of Little Rock's two major hospital systems, aligned with Catholic Health Initiatives, a national not-for-profit health system. This affiliation provided the financial resources that St. Vincent needed to help strengthen its market position, which was described as weakening at the time of the first site visit. The new financial backing allowed St. Vincent to take advantage of Columbia/HCA's exit and purchase the Columbia/HCA-owned Doctors Hospital and three family clinics. With these acquisitions, St. Vincent was able to expand its service mix and primary care capacity.

Similarly, QualChoice/QCA, a local health plan owned by the University of Arkansas for Medical Sciences (UAMS), improved its market position by aligning with Tenet Healthcare Corporation and other equity partners. Tenet owns four hospitals in other areas of the state and already has ties to the local market through its involvement in NovaSys Health Network, a statewide, provider-governed network. Tenet's investment gave QualChoice access to the capital it needed to expand its offerings and secure new business in the market.

Powerful Insurer-Hospital Alliance Held in Check

In 1996, the most potent force in the Little Rock market was the alliance between Arkansas Blue Cross Blue Shield and Baptist Health System, which joined forces two years earlier in a shared equity partnership to form what became the area's most highly subscribed HMO, Health Advantage.

Under the arrangement, Baptist Health provides the majority of hospital services for Health Advantage members in the Little Rock area, with the exception of selected pediatric specialty services provided by Arkansas Children's Hospital and services provided by certain hospitals in outlying areas. A similar arrangement is in place for the Blues' preferred provider organization (PPO) product. By 1996, Baptist's hold on this business gave it a clear advantage over its competitors. This partnership, and similar arrangements developed with other hospitals around the state, gave Arkansas Blue Cross Blue Shield added leverage to win managed care contracts.

While the Arkansas Blue Cross Blue Shield/Baptist Health alliance continues to be a dominant force in the market, key local organizations have begun to counter its power through their new associations with national partners. Through its affiliation with Catholic Health Initiative, St. Vincent has improved its financial stability and expanded its presence in the local market. The system bolstered its position by selling its 30 percent equity interest in another national firm, Healthsource. Despite St. Vincent's stake in the plan and exclusive provider arrangement with it, capitation rates under this contract reportedly proved insufficient to cover its costs. Thus, respondents note that the arrangement turned out to be more of a financial drain for the hospital than a competitive advantage.

St. Vincent has refocused its managed care strategy by pursuing nonexclusive contracts through the provider network NovaSys, which it formed in partnership with Tenet, UAMS and other equity partners in 1996. As an alternative to the Blues/Baptist alliance, NovaSys enabled local providers to join forces with others across the state to offer a substantial statewide network and compete for state employee and public school personnel contracts. NovaSys is now the largest provider network in the state, with 70 hospitals and more than 3,000 physicians. With this reach, the network positions St. Vincent and its partners to compete with Baptist Health and the strong provider network established by Arkansas Blue Cross Blue Shield.

At the same time, Tenet's parallel investment in the local health plan, QualChoice, appears to be strengthening NovaSys's tie to the plan, allowing it to bolster its position relative to Arkansas Blue Cross Blue Shield. Although there is no corporate relationship between QualChoice and NovaSys, the plan and provider network appear to be more closely aligned as a result of sharing Tenet as an owner. Since this relationship was established, QualChoice reportedly was able to secure favorable rates with NovaSys providers, allowing QualChoice to underbid competitors for the new exclusive point-of-service (POS) contract for the state employee and school personnel insurance pool. Though other plans offer products to this group—and Arkansas Blue Cross Blue Shield retains the largest portion of this business overall—the ability of QualChoice to secure the POS contract allowed it to more than double its enrollment and begin to make a dent in the Blues' hold on this business.

Physicians Move to Protect Income

Two years ago, while the majority of Little Rock physicians practiced in solo or small single-specialty practices, some had begun to organize into independent practice associations (IPAs) and larger group practices, marking a shift from Little Rock's traditional organization of physician practice. Attempts by health plans to adjust payment rates through profiling, coupled with the expected growth of managed care, heightened fear among physicians about loss of income and clinical autonomy.

As a result, Little Rock's physician market began to consolidate. Columbia/HCA's purchase of the area's largest physician group spurred other hospitals, including St. Vincent and Baptist Health, to acquire primary care physician practices and establish management service organizations (MSOs). Some specialists also moved to organize independently, leading, for example, to the formation of a new large multispecialty group and a loose affiliation of all of the urologists in the market. Hospital acquisition of primary care practices now appears to be slowing in light of concerns that these purchases have not yielded the necessary return on investment and have not increased referrals.

Meanwhile, specialists have continued to aggregate into larger groups and have found new ways to protect their income and clinical autonomy—primarily by establishing freestanding ambulatory surgery centers. The proliferation of these centers in Little Rock during the past two years has been remarkable. Respondents estimate that six centers are under construction, including those established by the large urologist group, Arkansas Urology Associates, and orthopedic groups such as U.S. Orthopedics and OrthoArkansas. At the same time, there continue to be some additional mergers of single-specialty practices; much of this activity appears to be driven by the effort to secure sufficient volume for these new ventures.

Many specialists view these activities as a hedge against fee reductions and loss of clinical control and as a strategy to increase their leverage with hospitals and health plans. Others in Little Rock characterize these efforts as an attempt by specialists to try to corner the market and retain traditional fee-for-service business for as long as possible. Hospitals view these ventures with considerable concern. Threatened by potential losses in outpatient volume, hospitals have sought joint ventures to establish their own ambulatory surgery centers with physicians. Both St. Vincent and Baptist Health have such arrangements in place. For example, St. Vincent established the North River Surgery Center in partnership with another smaller local hospital, the for-profit management company, HealthSouth, and a group of 40 independent physicians. While the development of ambulatory surgery centers is intended to bring physicians more referrals and ancillary income, the long-term impact of this expansion of capacity and potential fragmentation of the traditional delivery system remains to be seen.

Efforts to Control Costs Are Challenged

At the time of HSC's first site visit, some market observers believed that the infusion of outside players and the growth of managed care would help drive down health care spending and curtail excess capacity in the market. Since 1996, however, Little Rock providers have only increased excess capacity. In addition to the expansion of ambulatory care capacity resulting from the growth of ambulatory surgery centers, the major hospitals continue to increase inpatient capacity. Baptist Health and St. Vincent both are building new acute care facilities in North Little Rock; a new tower at UAMS added 100 inpatient beds; and the Arkansas Children's Hospital opened a new 50-bed neonatal unit. These activities appear to be driven primarily by hospitals' interest in expanding their presence in North Little Rock and the surrounding suburbs to make themselves more accessible and attractive to the residents and physicians in these areas. Since the repeal of certificate-of-need regulation for acute care services, capacity-building continues unchecked, despite the likelihood that these expansions will drive up costs in the long run.

Greater cost control through care management also appears unlikely in the near future. In 1996, all of the major HMOs in the market—and, to a lesser extent, the hospitals—had embarked on physician-profiling initiatives in an attempt to influence clinical practice and control costs. Plans were trying to implement payment methods that linked the level of physician reimbursement to performance indicators. In addition, one plan intended to use information on physician practice patterns to begin dropping high-cost physicians from its local network. Through these initiatives, the HMOs and hospitals hoped to move Little Rock beyond a largely unmanaged fee-for-service system, thereby bringing down health care costs in the market.

By 1998, however, plans had retreated from profiling initiatives in response to physician resistance. According to health plan respondents, physicians objected to linking reimbursement to profiling data and to the quality of the data itself. Implementation was impeded further by limitations of existing data systems.

Several health plans are again cautiously testing the waters with respect to profiling, primarily by focusing on providing physicians with comparative information on practice patterns, without ties to reimbursement. Arkansas Blue Cross Blue Shield is also considering a network-within-a-network strategy that would use profiling data to identify a subset of providers with whom it could develop a lower-priced product. However, the strategy has drawn mixed reactions from physicians.

Issues to Track

Little Rock appears to remain a market with few restraints. Although national firms have proved to be important partners to help local entities gain leverage, the threat that outside entrants would take over seems to have dissipated. Managed care arrangements have not grown as expected, but providers continue to position themselves for these contracts, while competing for the fee-for-service revenue that is still available in the market.

As HSC documents change in communities across the United States, key trends that bear watching in Little Rock include:

- Will alliances between local health care organizations and national firms remain stable and advantageous for local entities? Will these partnerships continue to allow local plans and providers to compete against the powerful Blues/Baptist Health alliance?
- Will plans increase their efforts—through profiling, payment arrangements or other means—to implement cost controls?
- How will the continuing expansion of capacity affect the cost and quality of care in Little Rock? Will the likelihood of higher health care costs spur purchasers or regulators to pursue more aggressive cost-containment strategies?

Market Concentration Increases, but Power Held in Check

The Lansing health care market has long been highly concentrated, and has become even more so over the past two years. Mergers have left only two hospital systems serving the community, and the exit of a health plan reinforced the strength of the remaining two plans. These few organizations, along with the community's three large local employers, share a balance of power, while unions and a strong local health department provide a check on their influence.

In 1996, there was tension among these major actors. Purchasers were exerting pressure to lower health care costs, and a proposed merger of a local hospital with Columbia/HCA was widely divisive. Key developments since 1996 include:

- Mergers have strengthened the hospitals while reducing capacity.
- Physicians' efforts to exert power have been thwarted.
- Public release of data on cost and quality spurred controversy, but purchasers continue to use these data internally to maintain accountability.
- The health department continues to lead collaborative efforts to reach underserved populations.

Recent Hospital Mergers Intensify Competition

Two mergers took place in the Lansing market since HSC's site visit in 1996, leaving only two hospital systems in the area. The Sparrow Health System-St. Lawrence Hospital merger in late 1997 brought together two local entities. After a failed merger attempt with Columbia/HCA, Ingham

	Lansing, MI	Metropolitan areas above 200,000 population
Population, 1997[1]	447,349	
Population Change, 1990-1997[1]	3.2%	6.7%
Median Income[2]	$29,999	$26,646
Persons Living in Poverty[2]	11%	15%
Persons Age 65 or Older[2]	9.8%	12%
Persons with No Health Insurance[2]	8.3%	14%

Sources: 1. U.S. Census, 1997; 2. Household Survey, Community Tracking Study, 1996-1997

Regional Medical Center (IRMC) merged with a regional system, the McLaren Health Care Corporation based in Flint. These mergers have left two financially strong competitors, reduced inpatient capacity and more starkly defined competition.

Sparrow-St. Lawrence Merger

In 1996, St. Lawrence was experiencing financial difficulties, and its physical plant was deteriorating due to lack of capital investment. Given overcapacity in Lansing hospitals in general and a declining patient census at St. Lawrence, it did not make sense to invest in much-needed upgrades. Its parent, Mercy Health Services, wanted to maintain a Catholic presence in the market and had been exploring partnership opportunities for St. Lawrence with Sparrow and IRMC for some time. An arrangement with Sparrow, the stronger of the two, appeared to offer the best option. St. Lawrence's strengths—behavioral health and aging services and its west side location—complemented Sparrow's services and geographic market.

The Sparrow-St. Lawrence merger was predicted in 1996 and is widely viewed as successful. Most St. Lawrence physicians reportedly have moved to Sparrow, where many already had privileges, although some chose to practice with the competing hospital system, IRMC. St. Lawrence has closed its inpatient medical and surgical services, but still operates an emergency room and maintains beds for psychiatric, substance abuse and hospice services. Community inpatient capacity is now somewhat stretched, and both Sparrow and IRMC have had to close their emergency rooms to nontrauma cases at different times because their inpatient beds were full. However, hospital respondents claim that reduced capacity has lowered costs for inpatient care.

IRMC-McLaren Merger

In 1996, IRMC was still working through the merger that had formed it several years earlier. While it operated in the black, it needed capital for facility upgrades to consolidate services and benefit more effectively from the merger. IRMC initially chose to pursue a partnership with Columbia/HCA, which would have brought the first for-profit general acute care hospital to Michigan.

While the Capital Area Health Alliance (CAHA), which at the time represented primarily the business community, initially supported the deal, four key market leaders—the United Auto Workers (UAW) and later General Motors (GM), Sparrow and Blue Cross and Blue Shield of Michigan (BCBSM)—opposed it. There was significant press coverage and public concern about the potential impact of this merger on IRMC's accountability to the community. Ultimately, the state Attorney General sued, and a Michigan state court ruled that it was illegal to comingle assets from a not-for-profit and a for-profit entity, thus preventing the merger as structured from proceeding.

BCBSM reportedly suggested several alternative partners for IRMC, including the not-for-profit McLaren, which was trying to develop a regional presence and which offered access to capital for IRMC. An affiliation agreement was reached in 1997 that made IRMC a wholly owned subsidiary of McLaren. Community response to this relationship has been favorable. IRMC has since improved its financial performance, increased market share and made significant capital improvements.

Since the mergers, competition between the two hospital systems has reportedly increased, even though both are operating at high occupancy levels because of reduced hospital capacity overall. Physicians report increased hospital efforts to align them to one hospital or the other through physician-hospital organizations. This trend may intensify if the hospital systems move forward with plans to develop exclusive products. Currently, both systems are exploring this option. The Sparrow-owned Physicians Health Plan (PHP) is considering offering Sparrow-only products, and McLaren is working on developing an exclusive network product through an arrangement with BCBSM.

Physician Efforts to Exert Power Resisted

Physicians have been uneasy about the concentration and power of Lansing hospitals and health plans, but efforts to establish their own base have been largely unsuccessful. At the time of the first site visit, several physician entrepreneurs were opening ambulatory surgery centers. GM views these facilities as duplicative of hospital capacity rather than as desirable competition and does not allow its health plans to include them in their networks. Meanwhile, the major plans have refused to contract with them, with the exception of PHP, which contracts with a center owned by Sparrow. As a result, the centers have been cut off from most of Lansing's privately insured patients.

In 1997, the Thoracic Cardiovascular Institute (TCI), a group of thoracic and vascular surgeons and cardiologists, negotiated a contract with Blue Care Network (BCN) to be the exclusive provider of cardiovascular care under a capitated arrangement. This would have given TCI significant control over payment for these services, putting the hospitals and supporting specialists in the position of negotiating rates with TCI rather than BCN. Sparrow and a group of competing specialists reportedly fought the deal, and new management at BCN withdrew from the contract. Had the contract gone through as originally structured it would have been the first of its type in the Lansing market.

Against a backdrop of these unsuccessful entrepreneurial ventures, physicians are adopting a defensive strategy of consolidating into larger group practices in an effort to counteract growing polarization of the market around the two hospital systems. To ensure continued patient flow if more exclusive network arrangements take hold, physicians want to have colleagues in their practices who can admit patients to both hospitals. As one physician said, "I could wake up tomorrow and find that Michigan State University [MSU] has shifted its entire enrollment to a different plan and that I have lost half my patients."

New PPO Gains Market Share

Well-connected to auto manufacturers and the UAW, BCBSM has a stable and strong position in Lansing, controlling well over half of the commercially insured market in the state. Until recently it had not been known as an innovator. However, the introduction of Community Blue, a preferred provider organization (PPO), indicates change, as it is a competitive move to shift enrollment from BCBSM's basic fee-for-service product to one that is relatively unrestricted and significantly less expensive. The PPO offers a broad network, an out-of-network option and increased access to preventive services compared to the traditional product. BCBSM is able to offer the PPO at a lower cost because it pays hospitals managed care contract rates rather than rates used for traditional products.

Early indications are that Community Blue will further bolster BCBSM's position in the Lansing market. It is taking business away from PHP and the Blues' own HMO subsidiary, BCN. Community Blue premiums are below BCBSM's traditional and HMO products, and in 1998, MSU converted all of its non-Medicare enrollment in its Blues' traditional and HMO plans to Community Blue. PHP lost enrollment to Community Blue as well, and was forced to lower its rates to remain competitive. Several other purchasers, including the Chamber of Commerce—the exclusive sponsor of Blues' products for small employers—have converted to Community Blue.

As a result of the success of Community Blue, BCBSM has been able to convert large blocks of business to the lower hospital rates without negotiating with the hospitals. Because they are receiving less money for the same population, hospitals are seeking recourse through the state hospital association.

Purchaser Alliance Regroups and Refocuses

In 1996, purchasers seemed poised to play a more active leadership role in the Lansing market through CAHA, the local health care coalition. The three large employers in the area—GM, MSU and the state—had joined with local providers and other health care stakeholders to reduce costs and monitor quality. The coalition became strained when its purchaser members began to exert pressure on local providers to drive down costs.

As a result, CAHA nearly disbanded before reorganizing and changing its focus to public health goals, including promoting wellness and supporting universal access to health care. CAHA has expanded from 70 to 108 members and has given seats on its board to the Ingham County Health Department, health plans and unions. The state has pulled out of CAHA, and the three large employers are pursuing their cost and quality objectives apart from this venue, with the state and the university working together and GM working independently.

One issue that all of the constituencies represented in CAHA can organize around is saving GM. According to news reports, the automobile company is considering whether to rebuild its outdated plants in Lansing or relocate them elsewhere. This decision puts at risk 13,000 GM jobs and an estimated 21,000 supporting jobs in Lansing. Demonstrating that Lansing is a good place to do business, which includes being a low-cost health care market, is a major element in the save-GM strategy.

Information Provides Mechanism for Accountability

Information continues to provide a way to hold Lansing health system organizations accountable to standards of cost, quality and community benefit. Efforts to report such information to the public have been controversial, so many of the data produced recently have been for internal use by hospitals, physician groups, plans and purchasers. The impact of this change on community accountability remains to be seen.

In 1996, the three large employers had a number of initiatives underway to gather and compare information across hospitals through claims data analysis. These led to a reduction in hospital rates in Lansing and were the genesis of additional efforts to look at cost and quality indicators across the hospitals.

Just after the 1996 site visit, the three large employers uncovered a substantial payment differential in what BCBSM paid the two hospital systems, with Sparrow's rates significantly higher than those of IRMC. Public release of this information was controversial and led to a reduction in hospital reimbursement and premium levels for BCBSM across the market. Sparrow objected to the process and outcome of this effort and has become mistrustful of additional collaborative information initiatives.

CAHA's subsequent effort to collect data on cost and quality heightened hospital concerns that the data could not be adequately risk-adjusted and represented only a limited patient base. As in many markets, providers are not convinced that cost and quality information can be conveyed fairly and accurately to the public.

Since that time, the hospitals have begun to produce their own data using a medical record-based system instead of one that was claims-based, to improve data accuracy and allow for risk-adjustment. The three large employers and the hospitals have been sharing information among themselves, but are not releasing it to the public.

No longer working together, each of the large purchasers is using data for its own purposes. The state and MSU have been analyzing claims data and are meeting with the hospitals individually to discuss the results; GM is using a health plan report card for internal scoring of plans, a system that may be adopted by Medicaid. But since these comparative data are no longer publicly available, smaller employers do not have access to them to inform their purchasing decisions.

Efforts to release data have also been pursued for the noncommercial population. Shortly after HSC's first site visit, the Ingham County Health Department released data showing that the level of indigent care that IRMC was providing was low in proportion to its overall market share. The report sparked controversy and ongoing disagreement on the methodology for calculating more broadly how hospitals provide benefit to the community. This issue still has not been resolved locally.

Collaborative Community Efforts Led by Health Department

The Ingham County Health Department continues to identify public health and indigent care issues and to play a critical role in bringing together health system and business leaders in the community to address them. Several initiatives to increase access are underway, and Lansing's mayor is playing an active role in these efforts, despite the city's lack of jurisdiction over health care.

Key among these initiatives is the newly implemented Ingham Health Plan, a program to provide coverage for the uninsured. The program taps into federal Medicaid matching dollars, bringing $1.8 million of new funding into the community to provide coordinated preventive, primary, specialty and ancillary care to about 7,500 uninsured individuals with income levels up to 140 percent of poverty level. Although the program does not cover inpatient care, funding flows through the hospitals as a disproportionate share payment. However, Sparrow has elected not to participate, which has reduced access to federal funding and limited the program's capacity. According to the county health department, if Sparrow were to participate, the program would be able to get an additional $1.6 million in federal funding and extend coverage to 3,500 more individuals.

To build on this program, the health department has also taken the lead in securing funding from The Robert Wood Johnson Foundation and the W. K. Kellogg Foundation for two initiatives to increase access to the uninsured. Access to Health will bring together local hospital systems, the business community, insurers and consumers to assess the needs of the uninsured and recommend ways to finance and deliver care to this population. Ingham Community Voices will provide funding to conduct outreach and develop an information system to support this effort.

Problems Looming for Mandatory Medicaid Managed Care

Enrollment in mandatory Medicaid managed care was scheduled to be complete in the Lansing area by January 1999, but health plans are having difficulty managing the Medicaid population, and there is some question about whether the plans will continue to offer Medicaid managed care products. Three plans currently enroll Medicaid beneficiaries in Lansing: PHP, The Wellness Plan and the McLaren Medicaid plan. Care Choices, the Mercy plan, agreed to exit the Medicaid market in Lansing as part of the Sparrow-St. Lawrence merger. Despite losses in 1997, the other plans have not dropped out.

Specific issues that plans have encountered in the Medicaid market include:

- Restrictions on marketing and automatic assignment for beneficiaries who fail to choose a plan have made it more difficult for plans to target healthy enrollees, leaving the plans with the potential for a higher-risk population.
- Despite a competitive bidding process, plans feel rates are too low, given additions to the benefit package and higher-than-anticipated administrative costs. They report difficulty keeping enrollees out of the emergency room and controlling utilization because of the lack of beneficiary copayments.
- Many specialists are reluctant to participate in the plans because the Medicaid fee schedule, which they believe is too low, is used by all the plans. As a result, patients are getting specialty care through emergency rooms or by having plans transport them to specialists in neighboring communities who take Medicaid. This is costly to plans and inconvenient to beneficiaries.

The Medicaid contracts run through 1999, but the minority-owned Wellness Plan is experiencing severe difficulty, and PHP has indicated it may drop its Medicaid product if it operates at a loss. The state is working with The Wellness Plan to keep it operating. If these two plans pull out, it is unlikely that the state will have sufficient capacity to support Medicaid managed care in Ingham County.

Issues to Track

The Lansing market continues to be dominated by a few large, powerful local organizations. Hospital mergers have created two strong players and polarized the market, and competition appears to be increasing. Unable to exert power effectively, physicians are organizing defensively so they can care for their patients in either existing hospital. The county health department continues to play a leadership role in expanding access for the uninsured.

As the market continues to evolve, several key issues bear watching:

- What impact will the increased concentration in the hospital sector have on health care cost, quality and access?
- Will physicians find a way to increase their power in the market, relative to hospitals, plans and purchasers? If so, how will they exert this influence?

- How will systems of care for the poor change, given the efforts of the Ingham County Health Department and health plans' difficulty under mandatory Medicaid managed care?
- Will early efforts to increase accountability be derailed given that cost and quality data are less broadly accessible?
- If GM does not rebuild in Lansing, what impact will this have on the health system and the local economy as a whole?

Integration Strategies Unravel, Competition Intensifies

In 1996, Seattle's once isolated and remarkably stable health care market appeared headed for transformation. The prior few years had witnessed the passage and then repeal of comprehensive state health reform; Seattle's largest employer, the Boeing Company, began converting to managed care; and health plans began contracting selectively with physicians. National plans eyed the market with new interest, local plans consolidated and took on a regional focus, while local health systems pursued vertical integration to compete for managed care business.

Since 1996, health maintenance organization (HMO) enrollment has not grown as quickly as expected, and several notable changes have occurred:

- Several providers abandoned efforts to operate their own health plans and revamped their physician integration strategies.
- The local nature of the health plan market appears to be eroding, as plans increasingly take on a national and regional focus.
- Competition among hospitals has intensified, with a new focus on developing specialty product lines.
- Turmoil in the individual insurance market and programs for the poor has left fewer plans serving these populations.

Managed Care Growth Falls Short

HMO enrollment and capitated payment arrangements have grown more slowly than expected in Seattle, taking providers and health plans by

Seattle Demographics

	Seattle, WA	Metropolitan areas above 200,000 population
Population, 1997[1]	2,268,126	
Population Change, 1990-1997[1]	11%	6.7%
Median Income[2]	$31,561	$26,646
Persons Living in Poverty[2]	8.1%	15%
Persons Age 65 or Older[2]	12%	12%
Persons with No Health Insurance[2]	8.3%	14%

Sources: 1. U.S. Census, 1997; 2. Household Survey, Community Tracking Study, 1996-1997

surprise. Although market penetration by HMOs rose from 19 percent in January 1996 to 29 percent in July 1997, it still remains below the average for large metropolitan areas and low for the West Coast. Meanwhile, providers estimate that capitation currently accounts for only 25 to 30 percent of their business, far less than they predicted. The popularity of point-of-service (POS) products in Seattle, as in other communities, may account for this in part, since capitation is more difficult to implement under these arrangements.

Several factors account for the relatively low HMO penetration. Until recently, Seattle's health care market was made up almost entirely of local not-for-profit health insurers and providers that have coexisted for more than 50 years. Purchasers and consumers have been satisfied with local prices, access and quality. Only the home-grown health plan, Group Health Cooperative of Puget Sound, had substantial HMO enrollment, and this still accounted for a relatively small portion of the overall market. Otherwise, purchasers and consumers favored traditional coverage and preferred provider organizations (PPOs). Because local health care costs and utilization were already low, HMOs had little to offer purchasers in the way of substantial savings, and Seattle's consumers generally have not been amenable to the constraints of closed-panel HMOs.

Despite this satisfaction with the status quo, dramatic growth in HMO enrollment was expected in the mid-1990s in response to new, far-reaching state policy and purchasing initiatives. In 1993, the state passed a comprehensive health reform bill that mandated health insurance coverage and was expected to drive most of the state's population into HMOs. However, major provisions of the act were repealed between 1994 and 1996, thus preventing this from occurring. Although the state moved forward with HMO enrollment for public employees, Medicaid beneficiaries and those in the state-sponsored health insurance program, the Basic Health Plan (BHP), there was no broad-scale conversion of the commercially insured from PPOs and indemnity coverage as had been expected.

Another anticipated driver of HMO enrollment growth came in 1996, when Boeing began providing incentives for employees to enroll in managed care products—a move expected to lead other purchasers in the same direction. Although Boeing successfully increased enrollment in HMOs from 10 to 50 percent of its work force, other employers have yet to follow suit, and the overall impact on the market has been more modest than expected.

Provider-Sponsored Plans Discontinued

In light of changing market conditions, a number of providers have abandoned efforts to operate their own health plans, due in part to administrative challenges and lower-than-expected returns on investment. Two of the major provider systems in Seattle—Providence Health System and Virginia Mason Medical Center—sold off their large plans. The Providence plan was sold to the local Blue Shield plan, Regence Blue Shield, and Virginia Mason's plan was sold to Aetna U.S. Healthcare, facilitating Aetna's return to the market. In addition, a health plan established by the state medical society in 1995, Unified Physicians of Washington, closed its doors after sustaining large losses. Finally, Care Net, a plan sponsored by the University of Washington and Premera Blue Cross, was eliminated when Premera consolidated it with other products.

While slow HMO enrollment prevented these provider-sponsored plans from achieving the scale they needed to be viable, they faced additional problems. Most of the plans were created to support the provider's primary business lines by acting as a referral feeder and increasing the provider's name recognition and geographic reach. But the administrative challenges of operating a plan diverted management's attention and resources from the core business.

Plan growth also was complicated by the fact that no single provider system possessed sufficient geographic coverage on its own to serve the broader Puget Sound area, much less the entire state, and securing favorable contracts with hospitals or physicians in outlying areas was difficult. Outside of downtown Seattle, plans frequently found few potential contracting partners, making it hard for them to obtain price concessions or influence care management.

Providers Reassess Physician Integration Strategies

The lackluster managed care environment—along with an oversupply of physicians and low prices paid for services—also has contributed to Seattle providers' re-evaluation of the ownership-based physician integration strategies they had been pursuing for several years. For example, Virginia Mason, a multi-specialty physician group with clinics throughout northwestern Washington and a hospital in Seattle, had pursued growth through acquisition of additional practices. However, limited returns on these investments and the demand for broad physician networks led the group to shift its focus to developing contractual relationships rather than purchasing additional groups.

Perhaps the most striking development has been at Medalia Healthcare, Puget Sound's largest primary care group. Medalia was launched in 1994 by Providence Health System in Seattle and Franciscan Health System in neighboring Tacoma. Amassing 45 clinics and more than 300 physicians, the group quickly gained favor in the market and secured an important contract with Providence's health plan for Boeing employees. However, Medalia counted on large-scale capitated enrollment to cover costs, a feat it was unable to achieve in a market that remains dominated by PPOs. The group's original business plan projected it would have four times the number of capitated lives by 1998 than it currently manages.

The pressures on Medalia came to a head in late 1998, when it announced a major reorganization. Medalia was divided into three geographic-focused operating units, reduced its number of clinics and established tighter relationships with specialists and affiliated hospitals. In Seattle, it signed contracts with the market's two largest multispecialty groups, PolyClinic and Minor and James, which give Medalia preferential rates, risk sharing for capitated lives and a stronger referral base—all of which is expected to help stabilize its position. While the effectiveness of this strategy remains to be seen, it is illustrative of the ways in which Seattle providers are now moving to adapt to the unexpected slow growth of capitation.

Plan Market Increasingly Takes a National and Regional Focus

Until a few years ago, Seattle was served primarily by a handful of local health plans, with 70 to 75 percent of the market enrolled in one of three local plans. By 1996, however, two national health plans had entered the Seattle marketplace, and since then three more have come in, gaining some market share from the three dominant local plans.

Because costs and utilization have historically been low in Seattle, it was seen as a market that outside plans would find difficult to enter. In fact, recent entrants have come into Seattle through acquisition or affiliation.

- Kaiser Permanente Northwest affiliated with Seattle's largest HMO, Group Health.
- Aetna U.S. Healthcare acquired Virginia Mason's health plan and, through its national acquisition, NYLCare's local enrollees.
- United HealthCare entered through its national acquisition of Travelers' small number of local enrollees.

Meanwhile, the two local Blues' plans continued to expand beyond Seattle, to the broader regional area. Blue Cross of Washington and Alaska, renamed Premera Blue Cross, has been marketing throughout the northwest, and many of the Blue Shield plans that had operated independently in each county in Washington and surrounding states consolidated to form Regence Blue Shield.

The emerging national and regional focus in the health plan market appears to be in response to the way the Seattle economy is developing. Boeing's recent merger with McDonnell Douglas has given the local employer a new national perspective, prompting it to standardize its employee benefits nationwide. Similarly, other mergers of local companies with national corporations—including Seattle-based SeaFirst Bank with Bank-America and Northwest-based grocery chain Fred Meyer with Kroger—appear to be pushing more employers to seek contracts that serve a broad regional and national employee base.

The influx of national plans has pushed local organizations to respond to new products and changing market conditions. For example, PacifiCare's entrance prior to 1996 severely challenged Group Health's Medicare market share by introducing a zero premium product. Group Health responded with its own zero premium product, which strained it financially. Group Health looked to its 1996 affiliation with Kaiser to help protect its position, but the impact of this affiliation remains unclear, and it is now reportedly scaling back on this relationship. At the time of the affiliation, it was thought that Kaiser would provide Group Health access to national accounts and provide the resources needed to improve its information infrastructure, facilities and overall competitiveness. However, some observers now question whether the anticipated changes will ever take place. While Group Health still accounts for the largest share of Seattle's HMO enrollment, it continues to lose market share and endure financial losses as it struggles with changing market conditions.

Insurance Products for Individuals and the Poor Are in Jeopardy

Health plans in Seattle, as in other markets, have experienced significant financial losses in recent years, and they have been especially hard-hit locally by problems with products in the individual market and public insurance programs.

In the individual market, insurance reforms, including portability, guaranteed issue, limits on pre-existing condition prohibitions and mandated benefits, have increased plans' costs. Meanwhile, the state has placed limits on plans' ability to increase their premiums. In 1996, Premera Blue Cross—the largest individual insurance carrier—sued for a 19 percent rate increase that bypassed state limits. Although it secured the increase, continued losses led Premera to announce that it would stop accepting applications for individual policies in December 1998. Seattle's other individual carriers, Group Health and Regence Blue Shield, have also sought regulatory approval to cap enrollment on certain individual products. Some carriers also have scaled back the benefits offered under these products, making them less attractive to those with higher health care needs.

Many individuals now appear to be turning to the state's BHP, which provides subsidized coverage for the working poor and extends nonsubsidized coverage to individuals at higher income levels. Because BHP benefits are more comprehensive than many individual policies, the nonsubsidized component of the program has experienced adverse selection. One of the most visible ways in which this has been manifested is in enrollment for maternity care. BHP is one of the few individual products in the market that offers immediate coverage of obstetrical and newborn care. This has become problematic for the program because pregnant women have been enrolling for this coverage and then dropping out of BHP after they deliver.

At the same time, the program has been beset by adverse selection—resulting from an influx of beneficiaries from the state's high-risk pool closed to new enrollees in 1996 subsequent to insurance reforms. Excluding maternity-related care, inpatient utilization rates for nonsubsidized BHP enrollees are nearly two and a half times higher than those of subsidized enrollees. Soaring costs have led BHP rates for nonsubsidized enrollees to increase by 62 percent from 1998 to 1999, following a similar increase from 1997 to 1998. By contrast, BHP rates for subsidized enrollees rose by only 9 percent.

Seattle's health plans also have had problems with the state's Medicaid program, Healthy Options, particularly with automatic enrollees—beneficiaries who have not selected a plan and who are assigned to one based on a formula. The lowest-cost plan receives 60 percent of auto-enrollees, the next lowest-cost plan gets 30 percent and the remaining 10 percent are enrolled with the next lowest-cost plan. Health plan respondents note that, as a group, auto-enrollees have higher than average health costs, which were not included in their original rate bids. As a result, several plans are pricing their products higher to avoid auto-enrollees; other plans have withdrawn from Healthy Options altogether. In Seattle, Providence reportedly had the lowest-cost plan until it dropped out of Healthy Options, leaving QualMed as the lowest-cost plan until it also pulled out. Elsewhere in the state, Premera Blue Cross and other large plans have pulled out of Healthy Options.

Plans' difficulties in Healthy Options and BHP are compounded by the state's joint procurement process for these products. The state requires plans to offer both products if they wish to offer either. Consequently, the decision to discontinue one of these products has meant that the plan drops out of both, although some exceptions have been made recently.

Provider and health plan representatives and advocates for the poor believe that many of the challenges faced by the individual market, the Healthy Options program and the nonsubsidized BHP could be addressed by technical solutions. Indeed, the state is currently debating options such as an enrollment lock-in for the BHP, risk-adjusted rates or incentives for continuous coverage that may help to alleviate some of these problems. In the meantime, respondents have expressed concern that the problems in these markets and the concurrent plan withdrawals are increasingly constraining choice for consumers, particularly the poor.

Provider Competition Intensifies along Specialty Lines

New pressures are confronting Seattle providers as recent alliances cause referrals to be redirected and as health plans squeeze reimbursement. Competition has intensified among area hospitals around key specialty lines, such as cardiac and cancer care. As a result, a more aggressive dynamic has emerged, and hospitals that were once praised for fostering a cooperative culture and serving community interests are now seen as seeking to enhance their reputation and market position at the expense of other hospitals.

Competition in cardiac care escalated in 1996 when Group Health established a jointly sponsored point-of-service product with Virginia Mason and closed its downtown hospital. As a result, tertiary care, including high-end cardiac care that had previously gone to the University of Washington, was shifted to Virginia Mason. The University of Washington sought to make up for the volume it lost by undertaking a cardiac-care joint venture with Northwest Hospital. Meanwhile, Swedish Medical Center wrested the majority of cardiologists from Providence Seattle Medical Center and established a new cardiac health management program to aggressively pursue this business.

Similar competition has emerged in cancer care services. Fred Hutchinson Cancer Research Center is launching the Cancer Care Alliance with the University of Washington and Children's Hospital. The alliance includes a jointly sponsored outpatient center and an arrangement to direct inpatient care exclusively to the University of Washington Medical Center and Children's Hospital. Previously, Fred Hutchinson referred inpatient care to Swedish Medical Center or Children's; now Swedish reportedly stands to lose about 9 percent of its daily census. New competition for cancer care also has come into the market, with the entry of national carve-out specialty management companies, such as Cancer Treatment Centers of America.

These changes represent a return to competition in core lines of business at a time when vertical integration strategies seem less assured of success and positioning for capitated contracting has become less of a focus. Under mounting cost pressure, hospitals have looked to secure key specialty lines to lock in referrals and income from this business. The new competitive dynamic that has consequently emerged marks a shift in how Seattle providers operate. Indeed, some respondents speculated about whether this competitive behavior can be sustained or will lead to some consolidation of tertiary hospitals or services in the future.

Issues to Track

Escalating competition and the entrance of several national actors in the Seattle market have prompted local organizations to find ways to protect and enhance their core businesses. As managed care growth plateaus, providers, health plans and state policy makers appear to be in the midst of a period of reassessment and adaptation. Several trends are worth tracking in this regard:

- What new strategies will emerge as providers move away from vertical integration? Will a new emphasis on exclusivity via contractual arrangements and joint ventures take its place?
- How will intensifying competition along specialty lines affect relationships among physicians, hospitals and plans? Will the aggressive pursuit of this business lead to some consolidation of tertiary care in the market?

- Will the local nature of the Seattle market continue to erode, given the growing role of national plans and ongoing efforts by local plans to regionalize?
- What impact will emerging difficulties in individual insurance markets, the Medicaid Healthy Options program and BHP have on health plans and beneficiaries? Will state policy interventions succeed in addressing these problems?

Local Providers
Fortify Their Position

In 1996, five hospital-based systems dominated the Indianapolis market. These systems, all not-for-profit, owned the market's most successful health plans. In addition, they owned or contracted with most of the area's primary care practices. Managed care enrollment was limited. Employers and state and local policy makers were not active in the health care arena.

With the 1997 merger of two systems, providers in Indianapolis have solidified their position, and the health plans they own continue to be the most successful ones in the market. Among the developing market trends:

- Provider systems are positioning themselves relative to the 1997 merger, so they can compete for managed care contracts with the newly consolidated entity.
- Single-specialty physician groups are consolidating, and the importance of physician-hospital organizations (PHOs) as vehicles for managed care contracting is diminishing.
- Providers are increasingly resistant to assuming risk in managed care contracts.
- Public and private sector decision makers are focusing more attention on managed care plans and their performance.

Provider Systems' Influence Grows Stronger

Several hospital-based systems have enhanced their already strong market positions during the past two years, in part to increase their bargaining

Indianapolis Demographics

	Indianapolis, IN	Metropolitan areas above 200,000 population
Population, 1997[1]	1,503,468	
Population Change, 1990-1997[1]	8.5%	6.7%
Median Income[2]	$29,851	$26,646
Persons Living in Poverty[2]	10%	15%
Persons Age 65 or Older[2]	12%	12%
Persons with No Health Insurance[2]	11%	14%

Sources: 1. U.S. Census, 1997; 2. Household Survey, Community Tracking Study, 1996-1997

leverage with health plans and stimulate revenue growth. Most significant, Methodist Hospital of Indiana and the Indiana University Medical Center (with its affiliate, Riley Hospital for Children) merged in 1997 to create Clarian Health Partners. This new entity has 1,400 acute care beds—23 percent of all acute care beds in the Indianapolis market.

In the three months immediately following the creation of Clarian, the two partners combined many administrative functions. Respondents reported that the post-merger integration of medical groups has proved difficult and will take time to accomplish. In some specialties, the academic culture of the medical school faculty has apparently clashed with the more entrepreneurial culture of Methodist physicians.

The Methodist-University union ignited some controversy. Competing care systems expressed concern about the potential market power of the merged entity, while community advocacy groups raised issues about the possible impact on the poor and uninsured. Publicly owned Wishard Hospital is closely affiliated with the University's medical school faculty and is the major provider of indigent care in Indianapolis. The merger raised questions about the future of this relationship and about the continued viability of Wishard as a service provider for the poor and uninsured. In addition, other observers feared that the merger would result in restricted access to care at Riley Hospital, which was widely viewed as a unique and valuable state resource for the treatment of children.

Since the merger, other provider systems in Indianapolis have launched several strategic initiatives in response to these changing market conditions.

- St. Vincent's Hospitals and Health Services, the major provider system in north Indianapolis, reportedly expanded its subspecialty pediatric services and acquired Lifelines Children's Hospital, a 21-bed acute care hospital providing rehabilitation and outpatient services. St. Vincent's also acquired a residential facility for the developmentally disabled. These actions reportedly were in response to Clarian's decision to increase prices at Riley Hospital and use that hospital's subspecialty services as leverage in negotiating with health plans.
- St. Vincent's also has strengthened its regional ties. The Daughters of Charity, St. Vincent's parent organization, created Central Indiana Health System, a collaborative group of hospitals in Indiana. This network is attempting to grow through mergers or affiliation agreements and to contract with health plans on behalf of its members.
- Community Hospitals and Health Services, which has three facilities in east and south Indianapolis, has extended its service area outside metropolitan Indianapolis by acquiring Community Hospital of Anderson and Madison. In addition, Community Hospitals continues to search for a merger or affiliation partner in the Indianapolis area.
- After a collaborative arrangement with St. Vincent's dissolved, Community Hospitals entered into merger and affiliation discussions with St. Francis Hospitals and Health Centers. St. Francis operates two hospitals in southeast Indianapolis, where the two provider systems have overlapping service areas. If Community Hospitals and St. Francis can reach an agreement, they may convert one acute care facility in this area to other uses. The combined systems would enjoy a strong negotiating position with health plans seeking to offer inpatient services in south and east Indianapolis.

Physicians Realign

A recent spate of consolidations among specialty practices has strengthened the position of some specialists in bargaining with health plans and provider systems. Although specialists in Indianapolis are realigning much more actively than they were in 1996, it is not possible to detect clear trends at this time or to identify common catalysts for change.

In 1996, the Indianapolis metropolitan statistical area (MSA) had 32 percent more specialists per capita than the national average. Today, small, single-specialty practices remain the norm. Typically, specialists still access patients through direct contracts with managed care plans, under fee schedules that have eroded over time or through subcontracts with PHOs.

Fees typically are set as a percentage of Medicare reimbursement; few multispecialty groups are available to accept capitated contracts.

In a merger that has drawn considerable local attention, the market's two largest cardiology groups combined in January 1999. The new organization, Care Group, includes 87 cardiologists, six related subspecialists and 52 primary care physicians. It is the largest cardiology group in the state and, reportedly, one of the largest in the country. Similarly, Community Hospitals' radiology group has merged with the radiology group at St. Vincent's and is considering another merger with St. Francis's group to form a single organization that can serve all three systems. Other recent single-specialty mergers in the market were noted in sports medicine, neurology, urology and orthopedics.

In contrast to the single-specialty approach, SpecPrime is a 350-physician, multispecialty network affiliated with Community Hospitals. SpecPrime contracts with a number of health maintenance organizations (HMOs), including Maxicare, HealthSource and HealthPoint, on a capitated, full-risk basis. It is currently adding specialists and expanding into adjacent geographic areas. Most market observers view SpecPrime's approach as an exception in the current market for specialty care and do not see it as indicating a trend.

Changes in the organization of physicians have had little impact on Indianapolis's primary care physician practices, most of which continue to be owned by provider systems or health plans, or remain closely affiliated with provider systems. However, many of the systems and plans that made aggressive efforts to acquire primary care physician practices in the early 1990s are now questioning the wisdom of this strategy. For example, Anthem Blue Cross and Blue Shield, the Blue Cross-Blue Shield plan in Indianapolis, recently sold its 250-member primary care physician arm, the American Health Network, back to member physicians. The network remains in place under physician ownership to represent its physician members in contracting with health plans.

Provider-Sponsored Health Plans Maintain Strong Market Position

Health plans owned by local provider systems, which dominated the market in 1996, have gained even more strength in Indianapolis. This stands in contrast to other parts of the country, where many provider-owned plans have struggled. In general, Indianapolis's provider-owned plans offering HMO and preferred provider organization (PPO) products have fared well financially during the past two years, while other plans, such as those owned by Anthem and Maxicare, have experienced financial losses. PPO products continue to dominate the market, although commercial HMO enrollment has grown from 19 percent at the time of the first site visit to 23 percent in 1997. Between 1996 and 1998, Medicaid managed care penetration grew from 35 to 41 percent in the Indianapolis MSA, while Medicare risk plan enrollment remained small, increasing from 4 to just 6 percent.

M-Plan, which is owned by Clarian, has the largest share of HMO enrollment; its membership grew from 122,000 in 1996 to 175,000 in 1998. During the same period, Anthem lost approximately the same level of enrollment from both its PPO and HMO products. Many respondents attribute this erosion to Anthem's lack of attention to the local market as it pursued regional and national expansion strategies.

M-Plan is now attempting to strengthen its statewide presence through a merger with HealthPoint, another provider-owned managed care plan. If completed, this merger would create a 600,000-member plan and a statewide network, with two-thirds of plan members located outside Indianapolis and enrolled in a PPO product.

With the exception of Maxicare, which has 81,000 commercial and Medicaid enrollees, national, for-profit plans continue to play a relatively small role in the Indianapolis market. However, CIGNA recently entered the market through its purchase of HealthSource Indiana, an HMO that serves enrollees statewide. Its ability to grow market share locally remains to be seen.

PHOs Become Less Important in Contracting Strategies

Providers in the Indianapolis market are increasingly resistant to assuming financial risk from contracting health plans, and, as a result, they are lessening their reliance on PHOs as contracting vehicles. In 1996, provider systems often used their affiliated PHOs to secure full-risk, globally capitated contracts with health plans. At that time, hospitals and physicians believed that they could control their costs and realize profits under global capitation.

Providers are now reassessing that assumption. Many are insisting that high-cost, difficult-to-control components such as pharmaceuticals be carved out of capitation payments, and that health plans retain some level of financial risk. Furthermore, many physicians are bypassing the PHOs and contracting independently with health plans to get some of the contract dollars previously allotted for PHOs' administrative costs.

Hospitals also see advantages in contracting directly with health plans. They believe they can negotiate better reimbursement for inpatient care than they can obtain under global capitation, where they need to satisfy the reimbursement demands of the medical staff, often to the detriment of the hospital.

Employer Roundtable Takes a Closer Look at Health Plans

Employers are beginning to take a more active role in the Indianapolis health care market, not through joint purchasing but through a collaborative group called the Roundtable, whose objective is to gather comparative information on health plans. Formed in 1997 by Eli Lilly and several other major Indianapolis employers, the Roundtable has issued a common request for information (RFI) to health plans. All but one HMO has agreed to participate. One health plan respondent suggested that by consolidating employers' information requests, the Roundtable's Rfi has already reduced plans' administrative costs.

Roundtable employers also have contracted with a vendor to conduct a health status assessment of selected managed care and fee-for-service employees. In addition, they have made clear their belief that Indianapolis HMOs should achieve accreditation from the National Committee for Quality Assurance (NCQA).

These initiatives represent a significant increase in activity by employers, which in 1996 were a relatively unorganized part of the Indianapolis health care market. Since then, health plan premiums, which had been stable for several years, have started to rise. In 1999, premiums are expected to increase by 6 to 8 percent for large employers and by 10 to 15 percent for small employers. In addition, employers have become increasingly concerned about the ability of health plans to manage care in a way that enhances quality and minimizes consumer complaints.

The Roundtable has brought together Indianapolis's major employers to address joint concerns regarding their relationships with a relatively diffuse health plan market. The initial focus has been on quality of care, care management and administrative issues. In the future, the Roundtable may serve as a vehicle for supporting care management initiatives such as disease management programs and reporting performance data. And although there are no plans to develop joint purchasing agreements, the Roundtable clearly could serve as a platform for addressing this in the future.

Legislature Pursues More Aggressive Managed Care Policy Agenda

State policy makers have been much more active in the health care arena during the past two years, particularly with respect to managed care. Like many other states, the Indiana legislature has taken a relatively aggressive position in enacting new controls over managed care plans, including requirements concerning grievance resolution, provider access, the use and distribution of formularies, coverage of new technologies and the annual submission of standardized information to the state. In addition, the State Department of Insurance has been instructed to review data from HMOs annually for NCQA's Health Plan Employer Data and Information Set (HEDIS) and release them to the public in a report card format.

Respondents suggested several possible explanations for this new legislative posture toward managed care, including a new governor who is more interested in health care issues, the concerns of a small number of influential legislators, the activities of other states and antimanaged care publicity in the national media. It is too early at this time to assess the impact of these new requirements on plans. However, it seems safe to say that health plans in the Indianapolis market will be subject to increasing scrutiny from the public as well as the private sector.

Substantial changes have also been made in Indiana's Medicaid program, mainly to accommodate the incorporation of the federal Children's Health Insurance Program (CHIP). Respondents reported that initial enrollment in CHIP, which began in June 1998, has been disappointing. Consequently, the state plans to expand its outreach and enrollment efforts.

New Programs for the Uninsured

The Health and Hospital Corporation (HHC) of Marion County remains the dominant provider of health services for the indigent in Indianapolis. Its flagship facility, Wishard Hospital, enjoys strong community support and receives $50 million annually from real estate tax levies; it also benefits from disproportionate share funding. During the past few years, Wishard has expanded its capacity to provide indigent services, launched an innovative managed care program for the uninsured and renovated and modernized its physical plant.

In response to growing demands for outpatient care, Wishard has opened three new community health centers since 1996. The number of visits to these centers has increased significantly during the past two years, even though the number of uninsured in Indianapolis has remained relatively constant. The Indiana University Medical Group-Primary Care, a physician group sponsored by HHC and the University's medical school, runs the centers. In 1997, Wishard launched the Wishard Advantage managed care program for the uninsured, with a benefit package similar to that offered by Indiana's managed care Medicaid program. Physician services are provided by the University's primary and specialty care medical groups, and Wishard provides ancillary and inpatient services. Uninsured Marion County residents and their families who are at or below 200 percent of the federal poverty level are eligible. Enrollees with incomes of less than 150 percent of poverty receive free care; others pay a monthly fee on a sliding-scale basis. In the program's first 18 months, inpatient use reportedly dropped from 800 to 400 days per thousand annually, and emergency room use fell by 30 percent. As of October 1998, Wishard Advantage had 18,800 enrollees.

Because of Wishard's close ties with the University's medical school and faculty, officials at Wishard were concerned that the creation of Clarian Health Partners would have a negative impact on their operations and on their relations with medical school faculty. To date, this has not happened. Instead, the merger between Methodist and the University Medical Center has forced Wishard to reevaluate its relationships with physician groups and the medical school and to consider other options for aligning with physicians. It also has led Wishard to explore alternative relationships with other organizations and to develop new strategies and programs.

Issues to Track

During the past two years, large provider systems in Indianapolis have remained strong, and some have even expanded their influence outside the city. The physician market is consolidating, as physicians try to enhance their negotiating power with health plans, but at a measured pace. Since 1996, policy makers have become more active in the health care arena, particularly concerning managed care. Meanwhile, large private purchasers have begun to work collaboratively to influence health plan performance.

As market developments continue to unfold, several issues will be important to track, including the following:

- Will there be additional provider mergers? If so, how will they affect physicians and their relationships with health plans?
- Will increasing pressure from employers and policy makers spur health plans to turn more attention to care management and to compete more aggressively on quality?
- Will locally owned, provider-sponsored plans continue to dominate the market, or, as in other communities, will provider systems move to exit the plan business and sell their assets to national companies seeking market entry?
- Will Wishard Hospital's new program for the uninsured prove to be a financially attractive and clinically appropriate managed care model for indigent care?

Ownership Changes
Set Market in Flux

Phoenix has experienced some of the fastest population growth in the country, attracting the entry of health plans, the creation of new facilities and the development of geographic submarkets for health care. In 1996, several potential changes faced the Phoenix market: two of the major hospital systems considered but rejected a merger, the area's public health care system was in a financial crisis, physicians began to consolidate and national for-profit health plans became increasingly dominant.

Since then, major changes in the hospital sector have emerged, as the two systems that considered a merger established other strategic affiliations. For-profit health plans have solidified their position, and although the public system has weathered its financial crisis, its future is uncertain. Other developments include:

- The market's largest not-for-profit provider system has been dramatically reconfigured.
- National physician practice management companies (PPMCs) failed locally, but physicians are seeking other organizational and entrepreneurial opportunities.
- New funding sources for the uninsured have emerged.

Large Provider System Reconfigures, Hospital Market in Flux

Locally based Samaritan Health System, the state's largest health care system, has undergone dramatic changes during the past two years, in the aftermath of a failed merger attempt with Mercy Healthcare Arizona, owned

PHOENIX DEMOGRAPHICS

	Phoenix, AZ	Metropolitan areas above 200,000 population
Population, 1997[1]	2,839,539	
Population Change, 1990-1997[1]	26%	6.7%
Median Income[2]	$24,911	$26,646
Persons Living in Poverty[2]	15%	15%
Persons Age 65 or Older[2]	14%	12%
Persons with No Health Insurance[2]	16%	14%

Sources: 1. U.S. Census, 1997; 2. Household Survey, Community Tracking Study, 1996-1997

by Catholic Healthcare West (CHW). Samaritan's reconfiguration holds potentially major implications for other local health care systems, competition in the health plan market and the future of the state's prepaid Medicaid program, the Arizona Health Care Cost Containment System (AHCCCS).

In 1996, Samaritan was Phoenix's largest system, with hospitals located throughout the metropolitan area. In addition to its 582-bed Good Samaritan Regional Medical Center in central Phoenix, it owned three hospitals in suburban areas, two rural hospitals and two skilled nursing facilities. It also owned Arizona Physicians IPA, the largest health plan contracting with AHCCCS, and cosponsored HealthPartners Health Plans, the only commercial health plan owned by local providers.

After merger discussions with Mercy foundered in 1997, Samaritan tried to solve its financial problems by solidifying its position in Phoenix's acute care market. Samaritan decided to divest itself of several components it did not consider essential to this strategy. First, it sold Maryvale Samaritan Medical Center to Vanguard Health System, a Nashville-based, for-profit chain, and its two rural hospitals to other buyers. At the same time, Samaritan expressed interest in acquiring financially troubled Chandler Regional Hospital in the rapidly growing East Valley and shoring up its own pediatric capacity at its downtown hospital.

In a second major move, Samaritan sold both of its health plans to United Healthcare, a national for-profit company. Then, in 1998, Samaritan announced its intent to be acquired by Lutheran Health System, a not-for-profit hospital chain based in Fargo, N.D., which at the time owned two hospitals in southeast Phoenix.

If the Samaritan-Lutheran deal proceeds, a national hospital system will, for the first time, become the dominant provider of inpatient services in Phoenix. The announcement of this merger has already had several significant effects and promises further changes:

- First, Samaritan withdrew its bid for Chandler Hospital, leaving the field open to competitors. CHW ultimately acquired Chandler, marking the first time it successfully affiliated with another hospital in Phoenix. Moreover, the affiliation gave CHW a foothold in the rapidly growing East Valley, where it could compete with the merged Samaritan-Lutheran system.
- Second, with the sale of HealthPartners to United Healthcare, other health systems are eyeing HealthPartners' 218,000 members as potential new business and are positioning to negotiate with United. If they succeed, Samaritan stands to lose some patients to other hospitals.
- Third, respondents speculated that United's acquisition of Arizona Physicians IPA could have a negative impact on AHCCCS.

Other hospital-based systems in central Phoenix are struggling to maintain market share, while those in the suburbs generally remain strong. Tenet Healthcare Corp., which owns four hospitals in the area, recently announced plans to pull out of Phoenix in keeping with a national decision to exit areas where it has not gained substantial market share. At the same time, Phoenix Children's Hospital, which currently leases space on the Samaritan downtown campus and contracts with the hospital system for certain services, is considering affiliating with CHW or pursuing a more independent approach. The county hospital system, Maricopa Integrated Health System, is also considering a major reconfiguration. In addition, the Mayo Clinic recently opened a newly constructed hospital in Scottsdale.

Collectively, the changes indicate continued upheaval in the Phoenix hospital market and suggest an emerging emphasis on suburban submarkets.

Health Plan Market in Transition

The dynamics of Phoenix's highly competitive health plan market are changing significantly in all sectors. In Medicare, new financial concerns stemming from anticipated slow growth in payment rates, along with the prospect of competitive bidding, are likely to intensify competition among Medicare risk plans. Meanwhile, the role of commercial plans in the AHCCCS program is in flux, and the privately insured market has become almost entirely the province of for-profit national plans.

Medicare. In 1996, the Medicare market was hotly contested, with competition focused primarily on benefits and provider choice, given high payment rates. Medicare health maintenance organization (HMO) enrollees typically paid no premiums and enjoyed extensive benefits, such as health club memberships. A high level of competition continues, even though Medicare payment rates have increased by only about 5 percent during the past two years.

Two emerging issues are likely to dramatically reshape Medicare managed care in Phoenix:

- Medicare payment to Phoenix health plans is expected to decline in the coming years, due to relatively small rate increases and implementation of risk adjustment established by the Balanced Budget Act of 1997. As a result, some respondents predicted that plans may scale back their benefits, particularly for prescription drugs, and institute premiums.
- Phoenix is a test site for a new competitive bidding approach to setting Medicare reimbursement rates for contracting health plans. If plans bid below the average rate set for a standard benefit package, they keep the difference in profit or can use it to add benefits to the standard package; plans bidding above the average rate will have to charge beneficiaries a premium. If implemented, this strategy could fundamentally change health plan competition for Medicare enrollees in Phoenix. However, there is local opposition to the project, and delays are already anticipated.

Medicaid. Commercial health plan participation in AHCCCS has shifted over the past two years, with two major plans leaving the market and one new plan entering. In 1996, some respondents speculated that several commercial plans had entered the AHCCCS market by submitting low bids and might not be able to continue to participate at such low reimbursement rates. By 1997, Blue Cross and Blue Shield of Arizona and Intergroup, an HMO owned by a national, for-profit company, dropped out of AHCCCS.

United Healthcare's entry into the Medicaid market through its purchase of Arizona Physicians IPA is an even more significant development. Arizona Physicians IPA has the largest number of AHCCCS enrollees in Phoenix and has won several awards for its innovative programming.

Although United has said it will continue to participate in AHCCCS, respondents expressed concern that it will not honor this commitment if its AHCCCS contract is not profitable.

Commercial. Phoenix's privately insured market essentially has been taken over by national, for-profit health plans; the only remaining local plan is Blue Cross and Blue Shield. By purchasing HealthPartners, the other locally owned plan, United Healthcare, leads the commercial HMO market. PacifiCare Health Systems, Inc., also increased its stake in the Phoenix market with its purchase of FHP International Corp. The Mayo Clinic, which launched its Mayo Health Plan in 1998 to compete in the commercial market only, plans to build enrollment gradually and is not expected to become a major player.

Physicians Regroup as PPMCs Fail, Specialists Consolidate

In 1996, two trends suggested an increasing level of physician consolidation in Phoenix: the acquisition of primary care practices and multispecialty groups by PPMCs and the development of locally based, single-specialty physician networks to contract with managed care plans. Since 1996, PPMCs have failed locally, but the growth of single-specialty networks has continued at a modest pace.

The financial difficulties that have plagued for-profit PPMCs nationally have been evident in Phoenix. For example, when for-profit FPA Medical Management, Inc., purchased the long-established, Phoenix- and Tucson-based multispecialty group Thomas Davis Medical Centers in 1997, it instituted several cost-saving measures. Physicians resisted these changes, and many doctors left. FPA declared bankruptcy in July 1998, and Thomas Davis subsequently dissolved. About one-quarter of the Thomas Davis physicians in Phoenix who had not departed previously left the state, and the rest formed single-specialty groups, started their own practices or affiliated with existing practices. MedPartners has disposed of its physician practices in Phoenix, while PhyCor, Inc., sold its Arizona Physicians Center to Columbia/HCA. Although the departure of these firms affects only a small proportion of Phoenix physicians, the failure of PPMCs has made primary care physicians less willing to assume risk in contractual arrangements with health plans.

Affecting a far larger number of physicians, single-specialty networks continue to grow, though gradually. These networks, most of which are locally owned and managed, provide a vehicle for specialists to secure capitated contracts with managed care organizations. Networks of cardiologists, general surgeons, orthopedic surgeons and oncologists are contracting with several health plans in Phoenix. In a relatively new development, five groups of hospitalists—physicians who specialize in managing inpatient care—have formed, and increasing numbers of health plans are contracting with them.

Taken together, these developments suggest that the consolidation of Phoenix physicians—as in other communities—has taken on more of a single-specialty focus, moving away from the primary care and multispecialty approach that once appeared to be growing more rapidly.

Hospitals and Physicians Struggle with New Relationships

Hospital-based health systems in Phoenix have had mixed results in their use of physician-hospital organizations (PHOs) to partner with physicians and increase their leverage with managed care plans. This strategy has proved most successful for systems in suburban areas that serve geographically limited markets and have greater contracting clout with health plans. Other PHOs have not fared so well. One started by St. Joseph's Hospital, CHW's flagship facility in Phoenix, folded after losing about $3.5 million in only two years of operation. Two other PHOs also shut down.

Respondents offered several possible reasons why these PHOs have had difficulty succeeding. First, many health plans have resisted contracting with PHOs, preferring to negotiate directly with physicians. Second, some respondents said that PHOs, which typically are led by hospital administrators, have failed to garner the trust of physicians. As a result, physicians view PHOs as negotiating good deals for hospitals but not for them. Finally, physician respondents note PHOs' high management fees as another factor contributing to their difficulties.

In light of these failures, some physicians are exploring other opportunities with hospitals—and independent of them—to shore up their practices and declining incomes. For physicians not in capitated arrangements, reimbursement is based on discounted Medicare rates, which have been stable at best or decreasing, especially for procedurally based specialists. In hopes of increasing income, some specialty groups are seeking joint ventures with hospitals and other entities. For example, three cardiologists have an equity partnership in the Arizona Heart Hospital, a new, for-profit facility with financial backing from North Carolina-based MedCath. Other specialists are pressuring local hospitals to build dedicated facilities and provide physicians with an equity share in these ventures and a significant decision-making role.

Some hospitals are responding, partly out of fear that if they do not, their physicians will defect. For example, Lutheran agreed to a joint venture with its cardiologists after MedCath approached the cardiologists with a proposal to jointly develop a free-standing heart hospital in the southeast suburbs.

Phoenix's hospital systems are struggling with the demands of their specialist physicians to develop and expand partnership opportunities. Hospitals do not want to cede revenues to physicians, yet they recognize their dependence on specialists for admissions. Many hospitals are attempting to expand traditional programs that favor specialists but do not require physician investment or risk taking—for example, by building outpatient facilities with favorable lease arrangements for physicians. Respondents noted that these types of activities have heightened competition among health care systems in specialty service lines.

Tobacco Tax Provides Support for Indigent Care

Phoenix has an important new source of funding for the uninsured. Under a 1994 ballot initiative, a tobacco tax was approved, with 70 percent of revenues targeted for indigent health care. Annual revenue from the tax has ranged from $125 million to $160 million. The tobacco tax revenue first became available in 1996, and $34 million was appropriated to indigent care. Additional revenue has since been allocated as the state's matching portion of Arizona's Children's Health Insurance Program, KidsCare, which began enrollment in November 1998.

Tobacco tax funds have been used to develop new primary care clinics, increase staff and services at existing health centers, subsidize care for medically needy patients with end-stage renal disease and develop a premium-sharing program for the working poor who are not eligible for AHCCCS. This source of revenue is particularly important because it is the only source of funds in the state to provide care for undocumented immigrants.

The uninsured population in Phoenix appears to be growing. In 1996, HSC found that 16 percent of people in the Phoenix metropolitan statistical area were uninsured; two recent local surveys reported that the proportion of uninsured was 25 to 27 percent. Even though the number of jobs in Phoenix has increased steadily, many of the new positions are in the service industries, where employer-sponsored health insurance often is not offered. Also, the decoupling of Medicaid and cash assistance under welfare reform reportedly has contributed to the growth of Phoenix's uninsured population.

County Health System Stabilizes Financially but Remains in Flux

Maricopa Integrated Health System is Phoenix's dominant safety net provider, serving AHCCCS enrollees and the uninsured. In a financial crisis two years ago, the system has stabilized under management by an outside contractor, but its future remains uncertain. Facing severe financial losses, the County Board of Supervisors entered into a management contract in 1997 with Quorum Health Group, Inc., a for-profit hospital management company. Quorum's contract was later extended through June 1999.

Under Quorum's management, the system is now profitable on a month-to-month basis, although the hospital facility continues to suffer from lack of capital investment. The reasons for this reversal are a matter of debate in Phoenix. Quorum contends that it has reorganized operational systems, negotiated more favorable contracts with physicians, developed new service lines and used the new tobacco tax funds to increase services to the uninsured. Skeptics paint a somewhat different picture. Some argue that the system's problems were not as severe as they initially appeared. Others say that Quorum has cut staff and programs substantially and instituted new and more burdensome cost-sharing requirements for the uninsured.

Even as the county health system stabilizes, a major reconfiguration is under consideration. The state plans to move to a competitive bidding process for the Arizona Long Term Care System (ALTCS), the long-term care equivalent of AHCCCS. Maricopa Integrated Health System has been the county's sole contractor for ALTCS; with this change, it expects to lose substantial revenue. In light of this and other challenges, the county is exploring several possibilities for the health system, including sale, affiliation, partnership with a local entity, extension of Quorum's management contract or negotiation of a new management contract with another entity.

This continued uncertainty surrounding the county system is a significant concern in Phoenix. Other health care systems fear they may be asked to increase the share of care they provide to the uninsured, while several respondents expressed concern that these changes may leave the poor and the growing uninsured population with more restricted access to care.

Issues to Track

During the past two years, national for-profit managed care companies have solidified their hold on Phoenix's health plan market. The largest local hospital system has undergone dramatic reconfiguration and has aligned with a large national chain. Other hospital-based systems in central Phoenix are struggling to maintain market share, and some have moved to position themselves in the suburbs. Physicians are seeking new ways to

organize and shore up their declining incomes, with an emerging emphasis on single-specialty networks and joint ventures. Bolstered by new tobacco tax dollars, the safety net for the uninsured in Phoenix remains in
place, but the uncertain future of the county-owned system is a cause for
significant concern.

As the Phoenix health care market continues to develop, the following issues merit particular attention:

- How will the Phoenix market be affected by the growing influence of
  national chains in the hospital and health plan sectors?
- What impact will the reconfiguration of the hospital market have on
  competition among providers and the services available to Phoenix
  residents?
- Will Medicare HMOs change their benefit packages and institute premium-sharing requirements for enrollees, in light of anticipated local
  changes in the program?
- How will health care systems respond to new pressures from physicians for entrepreneurial partnerships?
- What changes are in store for the safety net, given the uncertainty
  facing Maricopa Integrated Health System and the growing number of
  uninsured? Will tobacco tax dollars provide sufficient funding to serve
  the poor?

Market Calm, but Change on the Horizon

In 1996, the Miami-Dade health care market was marked by extensive deal-making that created expectations among local leaders that health plans and hospitals would consolidate. Meanwhile, high Medicare payments and relatively attractive Medicaid payment rates had lured many health plans to the market. Three major hospital systems were engaged in aggressive acquisition strategies, leaving the future of independent hospitals in question. The expected roll-out of mandatory Medicaid managed care raised concerns regarding the continued viability of safety net providers.

Since then, generous Medicare capitation rates have continued to fuel competition among the many health plans in this market. Although several hospital acquisitions have been finalized, there has been limited clinical consolidation or capacity reduction. Despite numerous efforts, few physician organizations have succeeded.

Among the key factors shaping the Miami-Dade health care market today:

- Hospital competition is easing, as hospitals solidify their positions.
- A variety of different physician organizations formed to assume financial risk, but many have struggled.
- Implementation of Medicaid managed care has proceeded without major disruption to the safety net.

Abundant Health Care Resources

Miami-Dade is a health care market of abundance, with attractive payments from Medicare and Medicaid, and an oversupply of providers and

MIAMI DEMOGRAPHICS

	Miami, FL	Metropolitan areas above 200,000 population
Population, 1997[1]	2,044,600	
Population Change, 1990-1997[1]	5.3%	6.7%
Median Income[2]	$19,811	$26,646
Persons Living in Poverty[2]	22%	15%
Persons Age 65 or Older[2]	15%	12%
Persons with No Health Insurance[2]	24%	14%

Sources: 1. U.S. Census, 1997; 2. Household Survey, Community Tracking Study, 1996-1997

health plans. The market, a mix of urban, suburban, ethnic and rural areas spanning more than 2,000 square miles, is economically and culturally diverse, with Hispanics accounting for approximately 50 percent of the population. The number of hospital beds and physicians per capita are among the highest in the 12 communities tracked by HSC.

This wealth of resources contrasts with the poverty and lack of health insurance in some of Miami-Dade's communities. One in four persons is uninsured, and the proportion of employers offering coverage is the lowest among the sites HSC tracks.

Public sector payment sources have had a dramatic impact on this market. The Medicare capitation rate ($763.19) is one of the highest in the country and has attracted many health plans. Despite exits from Medicare markets in other Florida counties where the rate is lower, health plans continue to compete for Medicare business in Dade, offering enrollees unlimited pharmacy benefits, zero premiums and no copayments. The Medicare 50/50 rule, which required all health plans participating in Medicare to have at least half of their enrollees in commercial plans, led to cross-subsidization of commercial rates, keeping them artificially low. With elimination of this rule in 1999, purchasers anticipate increases in commercial premiums. Furthermore, the Balanced Budget Act of 1997 is expected to moderate the flow of Medicare funds to plans and providers in the Miami-Dade market.

Medicaid also remains appealing to health plans, with relatively favorable reimbursement at 92 percent of fee-for-service rates. In addition, public monies from a half-cent sales tax in Dade County support care for the uninsured via the area's public hospital, Jackson Memorial Hospital (JMH), and its affiliated clinics.

Neither public nor private employers have had significant influence on the health care market, other than through price-conscious purchasing. The state's Community Health Purchasing Alliance (CHPA) program was launched in 1993 to help small businesses—a large component of Miami-Dade's private employer sector—offer health insurance to their employees. However, this program has not attracted large numbers of businesses. The Miami CHPA, with 3,550 member firms, reports that this failure is due to its inability to contract selectively with health plans, meaning it must take whatever price plans offer. One of the market's largest employers is the county school system, but even its influence is limited. Its recent attempt to drop one health plan due to poor performance was reportedly reversed by the state legislature.

On the heels of health plan fraud and abuse scandals in the 1980s, the Florida state legislature in 1992 mandated national accreditation for all health plans, and the state was an early adopter of an external appeals policy. Florida also has recently strengthened consumer protection legislation and mandated a report card on health plan performance. Because broad provider networks ensure consumer choice, purchasers are less concerned about medical quality and related report cards than they are about resolving customer service problems. Purchasers said that poor customer service is their top concern.

Hospital Competition Subsides

In 1996, the Miami-Dade hospital market was characterized by intense competition. The three principal hospital systems—Baptist Health Systems, Columbia/HCA and Tenet Healthcare Corp.—were actively acquiring other hospitals to increase their market share and lower costs. Baptist Health was discussing a merger with Mercy Hospital to solidify its position in south Dade and expand service to the Hispanic community. Both Columbia/HCA and Tenet were eyeing new acquisitions and affiliations to address gaps in service and market coverage. The future of the remaining independent hospitals was unclear. Several of them were considering mergers or other formal relationships with the three major systems.

Over the past two years, however, the high level of competition anticipated among hospital systems has not subsided. Two factors appear to account for this phenomenon. First, the perceived threat of Columbia/HCA to local not-for-profit hospitals dissipated, largely because its attention was diverted by an ongoing federal investigation. Second, hospitals have continued to pursue geographically and demographically based strategies to solidify their market niches, allowing them to carve out distinct submarkets and thus minimize direct competition. Tenet expanded its presence in north Dade through its national merger with OrNda and its acquisition of Hialeah Hospital and North Shore Medical Center, and it is now expanding north into Broward and Palm Beach counties. In south Dade, Baptist Health remains the dominant provider, with its ownership of Baptist, South Miami and Homestead hospitals. Baptist also attempted to expand its market share in south Dade through a merger with Mercy Hospital, a Catholic facility, but the merger failed due to differences over reproductive health and end-of-life decisions.

Free-standing hospitals have also solidified their market positions. Mount Sinai Medical Center's distinct geographic service area in Miami Beach has ensured its inclusion in most health plan networks. Pan American Hospital maintained its independence by strengthening its ties with the Hispanic community; it is operating at full occupancy and is profitable. The independent status of these hospitals now seems stronger.

At the same time, JMH, a tertiary care facility, appears to have strengthened its position. The hospital is planning an affiliation with Columbia/ HCA's Deering Hospital to increase its presence in south Dade. It is also expanding its primary care capacity by opening a primary care center two miles from the hospital campus and by contracting with primary care physicians in the suburbs. Together, these activities are expected to help JMH build its commercial and Medicaid business, increasing its paying patient base and its provision of more routine procedures, such as uncomplicated births.

In a related move, the JMH-sponsored health plan recently won the sole contract in Miami-Dade to cover enrollees in the state's Child Health Insurance Program (CHIP), KidCare. The expectation is that this contract will strengthen JMH's financial position as well by bringing additional revenue and referrals to the hospital.

While most of Miami-Dade's hospital market appears to be in a period of stability, JMH's expansion activities may disrupt this equilibrium. As JMH continues to pursue a more geographically decentralized approach and a broader patient base, the impact on Miami-Dade's hospital market remains to be seen.

Physician Organizations Develop, but Few Succeed

In 1996, most Miami-Dade physicians practiced in small single-specialty groups. The only long-standing physician organization in the market is the University of Miami Medical Group, a faculty practice plan with more than

600 academic physicians affiliated with JMH and Miami Children's hospitals. Hospitals were beginning to develop physician-hospital organizations (PHOs) and independent practice associations (IPAs) as vehicles to assume risk.

Meanwhile, the oversupply of physicians in Miami-Dade spurred national management companies and physician entrepreneurs to develop physician organizations. Most of these organizations, however, have been largely unsuccessful. Lack of information infrastructure, problematic reimbursement strategies and reluctance by health plans to share risk have thwarted these efforts, and many have proven to be short-lived.

National physician practice management companies (PPMCs), such as PhyCor, MedPartners and FPA, came to Miami-Dade over the past two years. But consistent with their experience nationally, these firms struggled in vain to meet physicians' financial expectations and their own bottom lines. Some have left Miami-Dade. Other companies, such as VIVRA, managed specialty networks for health plans. These ventures not only experienced financial difficulties, but also disrupted plan-provider relationships.

Hospitals, meanwhile, continued to develop and support several large PHOs and IPAs to increase their leverage with health plans and protect referrals. But this strategy won them few risk-based contracts, and hospitals and physicians alike seem disenchanted with these organizations. The Tenet hospitals are planning to abandon some of their PHOs and to reorganize their physicians into an IPA, but the implications of this change are unclear. DadeWell, a 600-member IPA formed by Baptist Health in 1996, has struggled to obtain globally capitated contracts, and it has not generated as much referral volume as physicians anticipated.

Frustrated by the bureaucracy of national management companies and the inadequacies of the hospital-sponsored organizations, some local physicians have begun their own organizational efforts. FemWell is one example. Its 60 physicians, who together represent about 80 percent of the obstetrics and gynecology business of Mercy, Baptist and South Miami hospitals, have banded together to contract with health plans. With just a 2 percent management fee, FemWell has reportedly begun to increase physician practice revenues and improve its position relative to health plans in the market. PhyTrust is another new entity, which manages globally capitated contracts with HMOs for participating primary care physicians.

While the future of FemWell and PhyTrust remains to be seen, physician organizations on the whole have struggled in Miami-Dade. It is unclear whether an effective organizational model will take hold in this market and what the relative roles of physicians, hospitals, health plans and national management companies in such a model might be.

Medicaid Managed Care Proceeds without Competitive Bidding

Two years ago, the prospect of Medicaid managed care worried providers and health plans alike. Safety net providers feared declines in their Medicaid revenues, as recipients were shifted from traditional fee-for-service arrangements to managed care options that might redirect patients to other providers (and therefore redistribute Medicaid funds). Health plans fought the state's attempt to establish enrollment levels based on quality measures, and blocked the state's plan for competitive Medicaid contract bidding.

The state now contracts with any HMO willing to accept 92 percent of the fee-for-service rate and meet certain quality requirements. For example, Medicaid plans in Florida must be licensed and nationally accredited, like commercial and Medicare plans. Having previously backed away from applying these quality standards to Medicaid plans, the state recently reinstated them. In addition, plans contracting with Medicaid are required to provide certain preventive health services, such as prenatal care and domestic violence services, which go beyond the scope of the basic Medicaid benefit package.

Nine HMOs in the Miami-Dade market were awarded contracts when the state began mandatory Medicaid managed care enrollment in 1997. Since then, Medicaid managed care has proceeded without much contention. Plans expressed little reaction to the decrease in reimbursement rates from 95 to 92 percent of fee-for-service rates; no plan has exited the Medicaid program.

However, health plan respondents expressed frustration about their administrative burden under the program.

- Discontinuity of enrollment appears to be the major concern for health plans. The high turnover in Medicaid eligibility and frequent plan switching make this a very unstable population for health plans, and the state legislature is considering a six-month lock-in policy to address this issue.
- Respondents also said that the state's decision to outsource Medicaid enrollment functions to an independent contractor has caused some confusion.
- Health plan respondents noted the difficulty of managing the auto-assignment process and meeting the program's reporting requirements along with other state and federal mandates.
- Finally, in the absence of competitive bidding, plans have no guarantee of enrollment numbers. This uncertainty, coupled with restrictions on

direct marketing, has left some plans with limited ability to manage this business.

Safety net providers faced a potential setback with the renewed requirement that plans serving the Medicaid population be commercially licensed and nationally accredited. This threatened the continued participation of safety net provider-sponsored plans that did not have the reserves or infrastructure to meet these standards. In response, a network of community health centers (CHCs), Health Choice Network, pursued an alternate strategy to secure and shore up Medicaid revenue. The CHCs formed a management service organization (MSO), Atlantic Care, to help manage the CHCs' Medicaid managed care business. Atlantic Care holds a full risk contract with the HMO, Physicians Healthcare Plans, for its Medicaid enrollees. Atlantic Care reportedly is up and running, with steadily increasing enrollment and a substantial return on the CHCs' initial investment.

In addition, under a special state pilot project, JMH has partnered with the North and South Broward Hospital Districts to enroll Medicaid beneficiaries in a new health plan with a more limited network that emphasizes more traditional safety net providers. The health plan is expected to begin operating this spring.

Safety Net Appears Relatively Stable

Implementation of Medicaid managed care does not appear to have undermined Miami-Dade's safety net providers, as some feared it would. There were scattered reports of some CHC service reductions as a result of declining Medicaid reimbursement; however, many safety net providers are working cooperatively to meet Miami-Dade's staggering burden of indigent care.

Because of its role under the Public Health Trust, JMH has been central to many of these efforts. JMH and its affiliated centers were designated as the sole recipients of the county's Public Health Trust funds for indigent care when the trust was established with the half-cent sales tax passed in 1991 and other local, state and federal funds. Although JMH's designation has been the subject of some controversy, the hospital appears to have lessened opposition to its continued hold on this revenue by affiliating with other safety net providers, including the Community Health Initiative of South Dade (CHI). JMH will provide CHI both technical assistance in financial management and short-term monetary support.

Partnership discussions are also reportedly underway between the Public Health Trust and Homestead Hospital in south Dade, which provides a significant level of uncompensated care. There is particular concern about indigent care needs in south Dade, where poverty and uninsurance rates are very high and rising and where, until recently, JMH has not had any facilities.

Meanwhile, several efforts are underway to respond to concerns about indigent care through a more community-based approach. For example, the Dade County Public Health Authority recently contracted with the South Florida Health Council to develop information on the health care needs of south Dade's indigent population and strategies to address them. In addition, Camillus Health Concern, a CHC for the homeless, is seeking partnerships with the Public Health Trust and other local entities to improve the health of the underserved in Miami-Dade.

At the state level, there have also been recent expansions to children's health insurance options, through a program known as KidCare. With funding from the federal CHIP, the Florida legislature broadened Medicaid eligibility for children and expanded the state-subsidized health insurance program, Florida Healthy Kids. KidCare is expected to cover an estimated 35,000 additional children in the Miami-Dade area.

Optimism about the expanded insurance coverage for children has been tempered by concerns about outreach and enrollment, especially for immigrant children. Even if the program reaches its enrollment targets, it will only begin to make a dent in the problem in Miami-Dade, where, according to HSC data, roughly 100,000 children—or one in five of all children—are uninsured.

Issues to Track

The Miami-Dade health care market appears to have entered a period of relative calm. Competition among hospitals has diminished as these providers solidify their market positions and the threat of continued acquisitions has receded. Health plans continue to be sustained by lucrative Medicare payments that, until recently, have cross-subsidized commercial premiums. Physician organizations have met with little success, causing some turmoil in the market, but producing no major change in the organization or financing of care to date. While persistent poverty and lack of health insurance remain significant problems, safety net providers appear stable.

Against this backdrop, there are a number of key issues to track:

- What impact will the elimination of the Medicare 50/50 rule and slowed growth in Medicare payments have on the market? How will commercial premiums be affected by these changes, and how will employers respond?

- What impact will Jackson Memorial's expansion have on the nature of competition among Miami-Dade hospitals? How will these efforts affect its position as an indigent care provider?
- Will an effective organizational model emerge that allows physicians to gain leverage in the Miami-Dade market?
- How will the community and state and local policy makers address the heavy health care burdens created by poverty and lack of health insurance?

Market in Turmoil as Physician Organizations Stumble

Orange County's health care market has undergone dramatic upheaval over the past two years, as cost pressures mounted. Area health plans have long delegated risk and medical management to physicians, leading to the emergence of large physician organizations that play a critical role in the delivery system. In 1996, physician organizations, hospital systems and several plans were implementing large-scale mergers to gain negotiating leverage and economies of scale. Between 1996 and 1998, premiums were relatively flat, despite increases in the cost of medical care. Because of the high degree of capitation, physician organizations bore the brunt of the cost increases.

Key changes since 1996 include:

- Two national physician practice management companies (PPMCs) filed for bankruptcy, and other physician organizations posted losses or downsized.
- Although Kaiser Permanente gained market share, it experienced its first financial loss in its 50-year history in 1997.
- Hospitals continued the slow process of consolidation, gaining some market leverage.
- Medicaid managed care implementation proceeded smoothly, but safety net providers continue to struggle.

ORANGE COUNTY DEMOGRAPHICS

	Orange County, CA	Metropolitan areas above 200,000 population
Population, 1997 [1]	2,674,091	
Population Change, 1990-1997 [1]	11%	6.7%
Median Income [2]	$29,703	$26,646
Persons Living in Poverty [2]	15%	15%
Persons Age 65 or Older [2]	10%	12%
Persons with No Health Insurance [2]	16%	14%

Sources: 1. U.S. Census, 1997; 2. Household Survey, Community Tracking Study, 1996-1997

Market Defined by Managed Care and Consolidation

Situated between Los Angeles and San Diego, the Orange County health care market is shaped, on the one hand, by being a part of Southern California, where statewide purchasing pools and large regional employers influence the strategies of health plans and providers. On the other hand, the vast geographic scope of the region leaves Orange County a distinct local market for health care, shaped by a strong local economy, a politically conservative environment and a rapidly growing population marked by ethnic diversity and economic disparity.

Orange County has extensive experience with managed care, and today it is one of the defining features of the health care system. In 1996, 46 percent of the county's publicly and privately insured residents were enrolled in health maintenance organizations (HMOs), compared with 32 percent for all U.S. metropolitan areas, and the remainder were mostly in preferred provider organizations (PPOs).

Even more notable, however, is the prevalence of capitation in the market. Orange County's health plans have delegated significant risk to physician organizations, typically paying capitation for primary and specialty care, as well as some ancillary services. Unlike many other markets, physician organizations in Orange County also typically share risk for hospital utilization and have responsibility for care management. While plans have broad networks, and most providers contract with most plans, capitation has resulted in tightly managed gatekeeping systems with clearly defined subnetworks controlled by physician organizations. As a result, consumers' access to care is largely directed by their primary care physician and associated provider network.

By 1996, significant consolidation had taken place or was underway in all three sectors of the market:

- Four of the major health plans in the county had consolidated, resulting in substantial concentration in the market. For example, after acquiring FHP International, Inc., PacifiCare Health Systems held two-thirds of the county's profitable Medicare risk business.
- A series of mergers and acquisitions in the Orange County hospital market concentrated more than half of the hospital beds in three major systems. As a result of its national merger with OrNda, Tenet Healthcare Corp.'s 11 local hospitals alone control more than 29 percent of the market's beds.
- In the physician sector, consolidation was also underway, with the formation and growth of several large physician intermediary organizations led by PPMCs and local hospitals.

Since 1996, all three sectors have shifted from planning the mergers to consolidating and leveraging the merged entities. Physician organizations pursued these objectives while continuing to expand as well.

Physician Organizations Squeezed by Cost Increases

While Orange County's health care organizations grappled with how to consolidate, industry costs began to rise. Between 1996 and 1998, however, premiums remained relatively flat—or grew by only a few percentage points—largely due to competitive pricing in the region. Physician capitation rates, likewise, remained steady, and rising costs hit physician organizations particularly hard.

In contrast to other markets where plans bear the brunt of these types of cost increases, the extensive use of capitation in Orange County meant that, in this market, physician organizations were financially at risk for delivering care under prepaid arrangements. Because physicians were often locked into long-term capitated contracts that did not account for rising costs, they had to tap into reserves or owner investments to fulfill this obligation.

Between 1996 and 1998, as in preceding years, physician organizations sought to expand the scope of their capitated services to increase their potential margin, driven partly by the belief that capitation rates for basic physician services were fairly bare-bones. Physicians continued to seek hospital risk-sharing arrangements, reasoning that good management of ambulatory care would result in lower hospital utilization and greater savings.

In addition, some of the more advanced physician organizations pursued capitation for pharmacy costs; others took it on, though reluctantly. Some physician organizations also sought global capitation—a consolidated payment to cover all medical services, including both physician and hospital-provided care.

As physician capitation arrangements expanded in scope, local health care costs grew beyond expectations because of a variety of factors:

Policy Changes. Several federal and state policy changes made over the past two years led to cost increases that physicians needed to absorb under capitation. For example, new legislation established a variety of mandated benefits guaranteeing coverage of certain services, which, according to physician organizations, led to considerable cost increases. Costs also rose with new requirements for physician-level encounter data for Medicare risk products and purchasers' quality and patient satisfaction measures.

Changes in Health Plan Offerings. In 1996, more loosely managed HMO products—such as point-of-service (POS) products that cover enrollees for out-of-network care—were gaining in popularity among consumers, who felt constrained by tightly managed physician networks. In an effort to be more consumer-friendly, many health plans also instituted new grievance procedures, which resulted in increased retrospective approval of services.

Providers reported that these arrangements drove up costs, while in some cases decreasing physicians' capitated payment. For example, under POS products, plans typically reduced physician capitation to account for enrollees treated by out-of-network providers. However, enrollees reportedly would go out-of-network for referrals, then come back to in-network physicians for treatment. As a result, providers reported that in-network utilization was higher than expected under POS products, leaving physicians with insufficient payment to cover costs and diminished control over utilization.

New Drugs and Medical Technologies. In keeping with national trends, local expenditures on pharmaceuticals and new medical technologies have grown rapidly. Locally, where many new contracts delegated risk for pharmacy, physician organizations had to absorb these costs.

Physician Integration Is Costly and Slow

While costs rose and revenues plateaued, physician organizations struggled to realize the expected benefits of consolidation. Integration efforts proved more difficult and time-consuming than expected, however, and the costs associated with consolidation exceeded the benefits achieved, at least in the short term, for three major reasons.

- First, physician organizations paid high prices for the practices they acquired. In competing for geographic depth and breadth, PPMCs and other buyers bid up the price for physician practices.
- Second, the cost of integrating practices, and the difficulty of melding the practice styles of diverse physician organizations, was greater than anticipated. For example, some respondents noted the difficulty of translating care management techniques across diverse practice arrangements.
- Third, the organizations needed to renegotiate plan contracts, rationalize physician payment arrangements and establish common information systems. New and often costly and redundant layers of overhead were added to manage these larger, more complex organizations.

There were some gains for a few physician organizations, however. MedPartners, a PPMC, and St. Joseph's Health System reportedly got better rates from plans for physician members than the physicians could have gotten on their own, and MedPartners had begun to consolidate physical space. But overall, physician organizations did not realize quick returns on their investments, nor did they achieve one of their major promises—the advancement and broad-scale dissemination of sophisticated clinical information systems.

Physician Organizations Falter

As cost pressures outpaced the benefits of integration, physician organizations faced significant financial difficulty. The 600-member Monarch IPA reported a 15 percent drop in commercial revenue between 1997 and 1998. And in 1998, the prominent Bristol Park Medical Group laid off staff and closed four clinics.

The most significant disruption was the downfall of the two major PPMCs, motivated largely by Wall Street investors, who, disappointed by poor initial returns, pulled out their capital. The demise of these organizations had profound implications for the market. They had purchased the assets of numerous physician practices and IPAs in Orange County and established intermediaries that assumed risk; their dissolution disrupted key arrangements for the delivery and financing of care.

The San Diego-based PPMC, FPA Medical Management, Inc., had grown rapidly in response to pressure from Wall Street investors. It acquired 600 physician members in Orange County through its March 1998 purchase of a large local medical group and its affiliated IPA. Only weeks later, FPA was in trouble—it was saddled with debt from its various acquisitions, had disappointing earnings and reportedly suffered from accounting and management problems. The company filed for bankruptcy in July, and by the end of 1998, it had sold all of its California practices and relocated its headquarters to Miami.

At roughly the same time, MedPartners was faltering. It experienced a failed merger with another national PPMC, PhyCor, in January 1998, and its stock value subsequently collapsed. By November 1998, the company announced its decision to get out of the physician practice management business nationwide.

Shaken by its failure to foresee FPA's financial problems, the state Department of Corporations (DOC) acted quickly upon discovery of financial irregularities in MedPartners' California operations. DOC intervened in March 1999 to seize control of the assets of MedPartners' risk-bearing subsidiary, MedPartners Network (MPN), to make sure that health plans' payments to the intermediary were used to pay providers locally and not to help bail out the corporate parent in Birmingham, Ala. DOC put MPN under a state conservator, who filed for bankruptcy on its behalf.

The Fallout. These developments raised serious concerns in the market about who is accountable under capitated arrangements for care that is paid for, but not yet delivered or reimbursed. Plans are holding physician intermediaries responsible, and providers who are owed money under FPA and MedPartners' global capitation arrangements—an estimated $60 million and $73 million, respectively—want plans to be held liable. The California Medical Association (CMA) has filed a petition with DOC to force plans to cover FPA debts to providers, but this issue remains unresolved.

The PPMC failures also disrupted physicians' contracts, raising concerns about patients' ability to maintain access to their regular providers. Health plans and purchasers moved rapidly to establish alternative arrangements with physicians to minimize the disruption and to protect consumers' access to their usual physicians. For example, one purchaser in Orange County intervened to ensure that its health plan would continue contracting with a physician group that had left the MedPartners network.

The state, however, has expressed concern that actions to protect plan and consumer interests could hurt efforts of physician organizations to stay afloat. Blue Cross of California attempted to transfer enrollees from MedPartners network providers throughout California in March 1999, but DOC blocked this action, fearing it would only undermine further MedPartners' precarious financial position.

MedPartners and DOC reached a tentative settlement in April under which MedPartners agreed to pay its debts in California and to continue funding its California clinics and IPAs until they are all sold. In return, the state will retreat from its aggressive oversight of MPN, allowing Med-Partners to resume responsibility for day-to-day operations. Significantly, the deal extends DOC's oversight of MPN to include MedPartners' California clinics and IPAs, which strengthens the state's ability to ensure that patients maintain access to MedPartners' physicians, and that physicians and hospitals are paid.

Long-Term Implications. California's increasingly vigorous oversight of health plans and risk-bearing entities is expected to continue. In response to the local PPMC debacles, new regulations have been proposed to increase scrutiny of provider organizations that assume risk; these proposals are expected to be considered in the state legislature this year. In addition, legislation has been proposed that would limit plans' ability to delegate risk for pharmacy costs to physicians.

The 1998 election of the first Democratic governor in 16 years also has raised expectations for increased market regulation. In recent months, there has been renewed discussion of either establishing a new regulatory entity or transferring this function from DOC to the Department of Health Services (DHS) to better monitor issues related to managed care.

Meanwhile, health plans have increased their scrutiny of physician organizations and have expressed a greater willingness to initiate corrective action when signs of financial trouble develop. On the whole, however, plans appear reluctant to drop capitation, and instead have focused on ways to improve delegated risk contracting.

Ultimately, respondents expect that physicians will feel the greatest effect from the failure of these organizations. Not only do they face potential financial liability for these entities' unpaid claims, but now they are confronted with the decision of whether to stay with the organization when it is sold, join another group or IPA or go solo. This decision is particularly difficult for physicians who have sold all the assets of their practices to the PPMC.

This turmoil contributes to a general sense of uneasiness among physicians in the market. Overall, physicians in Orange County are concerned about reported declines in income. Anecdotal reports indicate that some are retiring early, leaving the area or targeting lucrative niches in the non-managed care market. Several respondents suggested that physicians were more cautious now of physician intermediary organizations, for example, avoiding exclusive affiliations and refusing to share data with them and health plans. Moreover, physician organizations are re-evaluating their risk exposure, which could lead some to push for new contracts to reduce their risk for pharmacy costs and Medicare business.

Finally, respondents expressed concern about the implications of these developments for local care management efforts. Struggling with organizational growth and mounting cost pressures, physician organizations in Orange County found it more difficult than expected to focus on advancing and further disseminating techniques for managing clinical care delivery. As physician organizations evolve in this market, it remains to be seen whether they will have the incentives and capital to adequately invest in these activities.

Soaring Enrollment Leads to Financial Losses for Kaiser

Kaiser Foundation Health Plan, the local leader in market share, experienced its first loss, posting a drop of $270 million in 1997 and $288 million in 1998 on its business nationally, driven largely by problems in the California market. As a group-model HMO, Kaiser cushioned its physicians from the cost increases that other plans had passed on through contractual arrangements with independent physician organizations.

Perhaps of greater consequence, however, Kaiser also had continued its aggressive efforts to build market share by limiting premium increases. With premiums 5 to 20 percent lower than most other plans, Kaiser enrollment soared to almost 300,000 members in Orange County, an increase of nearly 30 percent since 1996.

This burgeoning enrollment severely strained the capacity of Kaiser's physicians and its hospitals. Kaiser has an exclusive relationship with its owned physician group and hospitals and referral relationships with a few contracted providers. In Orange County, Kaiser owns one hospital and leases wards at two other hospitals, but each of these was filled to capacity, so Kaiser had to pay high daily rates to place patients at other facilities. Moreover, the physician group absorbed the increased enrollment at a time when it was improving enrollees' access to primary care physicians, further straining provider capacity.

To reverse its financial losses, Kaiser abandoned its strategy of holding down premiums and sought double-digit increases for 1999. The state public employee purchasing pool, for example, agreed to an increase of almost 11 percent. The plan also increased its hospital capacity statewide to reduce referrals to outside providers, and it postponed opening two physician clinics in Orange County to reduce operating costs.

Kaiser expects these steps to yield positive returns this year and remains committed to its tightly integrated, exclusive group model.

Hospitals Benefit from Consolidation

Against the backdrop of market turbulence, hospitals gained strength. Like physicians and health plans, Orange County hospitals had consolidated in the previous years. Since 1996, they have sought to integrate to achieve operational efficiencies and to bolster their leverage in the market.

St. Joseph's Health System, for example, pursued physician integration through a strategy of purchasing the assets of physician practices and IPAs and pressing for increased exclusivity under these arrangements. This allowed St. Joseph's to consolidate contracting so that it could enter into "single-signature contracts" with plans that encompass all the services provided by the hospital system and its affiliated physicians. By bringing together several large hospitals and numerous physicians under an arrangement with increased exclusivity, St. Joseph's reportedly was able to gain better rates from multiple health plans.

Tenet took a different approach—contracting with physicians and providing financial support for administration, rather than seeking ownership of groups. For example, Tenet was negotiating a 10-year capitated contract with MedPartners, although MedPartners' financial troubles ultimately resulted in a more modest preferred provider arrangement. Tenet also merged contracting functions across its 11 Orange County hospitals, a move that helped some of its hospitals obtain new plan contracts but did not bring the expected gains in payment rates. At the same time, individual Tenet hospitals sought their own arrangements with physicians, in keeping with the system's more arms-length approach.

In spite of initial gains from administrative integration, Orange County hospital systems have pursued little clinical integration to date. St. Joseph's has had discussions about developing a common electronic medical record across the system, but these efforts are still in the planning stage. Tenet, likewise, has done little to integrate clinical functions, although it has achieved significant economies of scale through integration of some back-office functions and purchasing.

As Wall Street exits the local physician practice management market, hospitals increasingly may be looked to as sources of capital. Hospitals are in a strong position to benefit from the instability in the physician market, particularly as PPMCs sell off practices at much lower prices than they had previously. St. Joseph's, for example, reportedly bought FPA's large physician group and affiliated IPA for a fraction of what FPA had paid just months earlier. Despite the added leverage that these physician organizations may bring, it is unclear whether hospitals will pursue this business aggressively, given its demonstrated risks.

Medicaid Managed Care Proceeds Smoothly, but Safety Net Strained

Orange County initiated major reform of its health insurance programs for low-income and uninsured people several years ago, and by all accounts, implementation of these efforts is proceeding smoothly. In 1993, Orange County created CalOPTIMA, a semi-autonomous entity charged with developing and overseeing a mandatory Medicaid managed care program that relied on capitated contracting. CalOPTIMA became operational in 1995 and enrolled all recipients eligible through their receipt of cash assistance, as well as those eligible under programs for the aged and disabled. CalOPTIMA has won praise for expanding access to providers; currently, 85 percent of the county's physicians now see Medi-Cal enrollees.

Through new contracts executed in 1998, the program is increasing its attention to clinical care management and quality improvement. CalOPTIMA purchases services for its Medi-Cal members via capitated contracts with health plans or physician-hospital consortia (PHCs) created specially for the program. New contracts changed the payment split between hospitals and physicians in favor of physicians, and altered physician-hospital risk-sharing arrangements begun in 1995 to reduce hospitalizations and increase coordination between physicians and hospitals.

CalOPTIMA also is raising the minimum number of enrollees for PHCs and health plans from 2,500 to 5,000 in an effort to reduce administrative burden to the participating plans and the program overall. This is intended to allow for a greater focus on quality improvement and to help plans manage enrollment declines due to welfare reform and improvements in the local economy. CalOPTIMA's enrollment of people eligible through cash assistance programs has declined 30 percent since 1995.

Safety Net Providers. From its inception, CalOPTIMA took steps to ensure the participation of traditional safety net providers, but began contracting with plans and PHCs that included other hospitals and physicians as well. There is no public hospital in the county, and two hospitals—the University of California at Irvine Medical Center (UCIMC) and Children's Hospital of Orange County (CHOC)—serve as the county's major safety net hospitals. CalOPTIMA has attempted to support these and other safety net providers by favoring PHCs that include them in the assignment of members who do not select a plan voluntarily.

While UCIMC's PHC has shown signs of enrollment growth recently, both safety net hospitals are now under significant financial pressure because many Medi-Cal beneficiaries enroll in other plans and PHCs that have broader geographic networks. UCIMC is seeking to increase its commercial patients to offset its declining Medi-Cal patient base, although commercial payments are also under pressure. CHOC received an influx of Medicaid disproportionate share funds between 1996 and 1998; however, the loss of the Medi-Cal volume puts those funds at risk at both hospitals.

Complicating matters for CHOC, local hospitals began charging lower prices for advanced pediatric care. As a result, commercial plans were lured away from CHOC, and the hospital's occupancy rate dropped to 30 percent. It subsequently reduced staffing considerably, consolidated admissions and some administrative functions with neighboring St. Joseph's and closed a clinic. Meanwhile, UCIMC also has cut back staffing, even though emergency room visits by indigent persons have increased and UCIMC-affiliated specialists at three community clinics are reportedly experiencing great increases in demand. UCIMC is one of few places in the county that provides free follow-up care with specialists for the indigent population.

Care for the Medically Indigent. Responsibility for care for the medically indigent remains the subject of much debate in Orange County. From the beginning, CalOPTIMA was slated to take over the county's program for the medically indigent, Medical Services for the Indigent (MSI). Under California law, counties are responsible for providing care to the medically indigent; they use a mix of state revenues and their own funds to support this care. Despite recent small increases to specialists, annual funding is fixed, and the program reportedly reimburses providers for less than one-fifth of the cost of providers' billed charges. While MSI has contributed to the cost of care for 20,000 indigent patients with medical need, this constitutes only a fraction of the estimated 335,000 uninsured adults in the county.

CalOPTIMA has been hesitant to take over MSI, wary of the overall financial implications of this responsibility and the lack of information about the size of this population and its health needs. CalOPTIMA and the county are now working on a pilot managed care program to develop data on costs and clinical care requirements as a way to consider these issues more carefully. The county also recently stepped up eligibility verification standards to better ensure that the program focuses on its intended population—a move that is expected to limit MSI enrollment.

Advocates for the poor remain concerned about the ability of the safety net to provide care to Orange County's uninsured immigrant population, which continues to grow, particularly among Hispanics and Southeast Asians. Initiatives are underway to better serve this population, including a new community health center (CHC) serving Vietnamese immigrants and additional federal and grant funding for local CHCs.

However, many people in the county who need health care remain outside the mainstream of services, including immigrants, who may fear that using the public system could result in their deportation. This fear, as well as other cultural and socioeconomic barriers to care, has fueled reliance on so-called back office clinics where unlicensed individuals provide health care and distribute pharmaceuticals illegally. Recently, two children who were treated in unlicensed clinics died. County officials are exploring how to adapt the existing safety net to better serve the diverse populations in need of health care services.

Issues to Track

Many of the features of this mature managed care market appear to be fraying under financial pressures and consumer demands for more loosely managed insurance products. Integration efforts have been slow and costly for hospitals and physicians, and the high-profile failure of several large physician organizations and difficulties of others present serious challenges to a delivery system built on capitation and tight networks. Regulatory bodies are stepping up their scrutiny of risk relationships, and state policy changes appear likely.

The cost pressures that physicians have faced over the past two years remain and may intensify in the next few years. Additional benefit mandates and managed care regulations are expected from the state legislature, and decreasing Medicare payments under the Balanced Budget Act of 1997 will further constrain revenue for plans and providers.

However, health plans are raising premiums now and appear to be getting higher-than-historical increases in the short term. It remains to be seen whether premium increases will result in large enough payments to physician organizations to offset the severe financial pressures that confronted them over the past few years. In this environment, several other issues bear watching:

- How will physician organizations emerge from this turmoil? Where will physicians displaced by the exit of MedPartners go? Will hospitals begin to play a larger role in financing and leading physician organizations, and, if so, will this lead to greater exclusivity?
- How will delegation of financial risk and care management evolve in this market? What impact will these changes have on the development and dissemination of clinical information systems and techniques to improve clinical care?
- How will policy makers reshape the way they monitor entities that assume financial risk for health care delivery?

- How will employers react to premium increases, and what impact will this have on consumers? Will the business community begin to lobby against managed care regulation or seek other ways to control health care costs?
- Will the county and CalOPTIMA find a mutually acceptable model for managed care for the uninsured? How will safety net providers fare in light of continued pressures from competition for Medicaid patients?

Competition Intensifies
after Proposed Merger Fails

Intense competition among hospital-based systems continues to characterize the Greenville health care market after a proposed merger between three major hospitals failed because of public opposition in 1997. Today, hospitals continue to compete in three historically distinct submarkets. However, some are also targeting an area of rapid economic growth outside of their traditional specific areas. Meanwhile, hospital systems are continuing to develop the infrastructure both to accept risk and manage the physician practices they aggressively acquired. But given the tight labor market, employers remain less concerned with constraining costs, and more with offering broad provider networks. As a result, enrollment growth in health maintenance organizations (HMOs) has been slower than expected. Among the major trends shaping the Greenville health care market today:

- Health plans' interest in risk-based contracts with providers has diminished.
- Hospital systems have implemented productivity-based payment for physicians and expanded clinical care management efforts.
- Despite improvements to the safety net, gaps remain.

Hospital Competition Escalates in Light of Failed Merger

The Greenville market, which encompasses a five-county area in the upstate region of South Carolina, continues to be noted for significant economic growth. Multinational companies such as BMW and Michelin are contributing to this expanding economic base, creating a tight labor

GREENVILLE DEMOGRAPHICS

	Greenville, SC	Metropolitan areas above 200,000 population
Population, 1997[1]	904,729	
Population Change, 1990-1997[1]	8.5%	6.7%
Median Income[2]	$23,605	$26,646
Persons Living in Poverty[2]	15%	15%
Persons Age 65 or Older[2]	13%	12%
Persons with No Health Insurance[2]	12%	14%

Sources: 1. U.S. Census, 1997; 2. Household Survey, Community Tracking Study, 1996-1997

market. Population in the area increased at a rate of 8.5 percent between 1990 and 1997, and unemployment is only 1.8 percent.

Three concentrated and distinct submarkets for health care center around Greenville, Spartanburg and Anderson counties, with some overlap in the area between Greenville and Spartanburg, where economic growth has been most rapid.

- Greenville County is home to the largest health care institution in the market, Greenville Hospital System (GHS). GHS controls 75 percent of inpatient services in the county and is the area's only teaching hospital. Also in Greenville County, St. Francis Health System is GHS's major local competitor. The two systems have a long-standing rivalry, with GHS offering discounts to health plans that exclude St. Francis from their networks. At the time of HSC's first site visit, St. Francis had opened a women's hospital in the area between Greenville and Spartanburg, and GHS quickly bought up the property surrounding it.
- In Spartanburg County, the largest hospital system is Spartanburg Regional Healthcare System. Its chief competitor, Mary Black Memorial Hospital, is owned by Quorum Health Group, a national hospital chain. Spartanburg Regional is the major tertiary care provider in the county and accounts for 70 percent of inpatient care in Spartanburg County.
- Anderson Area Medical Center is the sole hospital system serving Anderson County.

Despite the distinctiveness of each of these submarkets, large companies, which account for more than half of the local work force, draw their employees from the entire region. As a result, employers are demanding that health plans offer provider networks that can serve residents in all three areas.

In 1995, GHS, Spartanburg Regional and Anderson Area Medical Center proposed merging into a single system, known as AGS, that would span the Greenville market's three major counties. The new provider entity sought economies of scale in operations and information systems and a strong negotiating position with insurers. It also would have appealed to plans seeking a single, geographically dispersed provider network to serve large regional employers.

Within the Greenville community, opposition to the merger emerged amid fears that local control over health care would be lost to a monopoly controlled by GHS. Community distrust of GHS, fueled in part by a marketing campaign spearheaded by St. Francis, culminated in a 1996 referendum in which 75 percent of voters rejected the merger proposal. Although the referendum was nonbinding, the message sent by voters was so strong that GHS decided to pull out of the deal and repair its relations with the community.

After the AGS merger fell apart, local hospitals sought to solidify and improve their position relative to competitors, both in their immediate submarkets and in the market as a whole. In Greenville County, St. Francis stepped up its strategy to capture market share from GHS by broadening its subspecialty service mix and marketing itself as a patient-friendly hospital offering a range of services comparable to those of GHS. St. Francis recently received certificate-of-need (CON) approval from the state to offer open-heart surgery, which several plans, including Blue Cross and Blue Shield of South Carolina and CIGNA/Healthsource, had said was necessary if they were to include St. Francis in their networks. But despite several large purchasers' special appeals to one of these plans, both continue to exclude the hospital from their networks because of the steep discount offered by GHS.

GHS and its former AGS partners continue to participate in certain activities begun in expectation of the merger, including the joint ownership of a health plan, HealthFirst, created largely in anticipation of mandatory Medicaid managed care. At the same time, however, Spartanburg Regional and Anderson Area Medical have moved to strengthen their positions as tertiary care providers. Anderson has applied for a CON to perform open-heart surgery, and Spartanburg is currently building a cancer center.

Meanwhile, competition for the expanding health care market between Greenville and Spartanburg has intensified, reflecting the emergence of direct competition among hospitals that had long confined their service areas to more narrowly defined submarkets. GHS is now completing a large ambulatory surgery and physician office complex in this strategic area, on the property surrounding St. Francis's women's hospital. Spartanburg Regional has established pediatric and orthopedic physician practices and family care centers. At the same time, Mary Black Memorial has placed obstetrics-gynecology practices in this demographically desirable area. Hospitals also have built urgent care centers and are marketing their occupational health services to employers based there.

Two recent market developments point to potential further changes in Greenville hospitals' competitive environment. First, it was recently announced that St. Francis Health System is up for sale, as its owner, the Franciscan Sisters of the Poor Health System, decided to leave the health care business on the heels of losses in other markets. A change in ownership of this hospital could affect the market position or strategies of St. Francis, altering competition in Greenville County and in the market at large.

Second, Spartanburg Regional recently agreed to consider joint venture opportunities with Charlotte, N.C.-based Carolina Medical System. Respondent reactions to this announcement were mixed. Since no joint ventures have been identified yet, some respondents indicated that it was too soon to assess the implications of this arrangement. Others noted, however, that if Spartanburg moves forward with these activities, it will give an organization from an adjacent market an important foothold in the area and may lead to more regionally based competition.

Plans Back Away from Provider Risk Contracting

At the time of the first site visit in 1997, HMO enrollment was limited, but it was expected to increase. National plans such as CIGNA/HealthSource and Aetna had established a strong presence in the market. With half of the insured work force enrolled in preferred provider organizations (PPOs), an ongoing transition into HMOs and more restrictive provider networks was anticipated. Plans had begun to establish risk-based contracts with providers, which also were expected to grow.

Two years later, however, HMO enrollment has increased more modestly than expected, as employers remain reluctant to usher employees into more restrictive products. Greenville continues to have the lowest HMO penetration of the 12 communities HSC tracks.

At the same time, health plans' interest in risk-contracting arrangements with providers has diminished. Maxicare, a national plan, had established capitated contracts with hospitals, but has since left this market after failing to recover from its national bankruptcy in the 1980s. Blue Cross and Blue Shield, the leading health plan with respect to market share, has several capitated contracts, yet it has found that improved utilization review techniques have enabled it to rein in costs more effectively through dis-counted fee-for-service. As a result, its fee-for-service arrangements are now less costly than its capitated contracts, and it is reportedly less inclined toward capitation for future contracts.

Meanwhile, HealthFirst, the health plan formed by the AGS partners, has established itself as an independent competitor among health plans in the market, expanding well beyond its role as a vehicle for AGS partners to accept risk. Over the past two years, HealthFirst's enrollment has increased substantially, its product offerings have broadened and it is expected to yield a profit for the first time in 1999. In the wake of the failed merger, the hospital owners now appear to view the plan primarily as an investment rather than as a vehicle for shared risk contracting.

Other provider-initiated efforts at risk contracting have also been un-successful. The multispecialty group, Carolina Multispecialty Associates (CMA), noted two years ago for its aggressive move to organize physicians in anticipation of managed care, has dissolved. At the time of the first site visit, CMA was rapidly building its management infrastructure, and was actively seeking capitated contracts. Both GHS and St. Francis expressed interest then in purchasing this emergent competitor. But when risk con-tracting failed to materialize, CMA physicians were less inclined to support costly information and contracting systems with dim prospects for returns on these investments. Starting with cardiologists, specialists began leaving CMA, its ranks shrinking from 75 physicians to 45 before it dissolved.

CMA's demise presents a striking example of failed expectations of change in the Greenville market. In 1997, market observers noted CMA as the organization most likely to manage full-risk capitation contracts, and, as such, it represented a potential physician-led challenge to a market his-torically dominated by hospital-based systems. CMA's failure reflects the lack of change in the underlying market conditions in Greenville, as fee-for-service payment and the unrivaled leadership of hospital-based systems continue to prevail.

Hospitals Continue to Pursue Integration

Despite the movement away from risk-based contracting, hospitals have continued their efforts to develop the infrastructure necessary for these ar-rangements. In 1997, hospitals were continuing an aggressive campaign to acquire primary care practices. Ultimately, almost 75 percent of the area's primary care physicians came under the ownership of local hospitals—more than in any other HSC study site. Integration was limited, however, because hospitals did not have the information systems to monitor cost and quality.

Two years later, hospitals have taken steps toward integration by strengthening their information systems and establishing profiling systems to monitor physician practice patterns. A significant reduction in length of stay across most diagnosis-related groups (DRGs) at a number of local hospitals was attributed to hospital-initiated physician profiling efforts.

In addition, the hospitals are beginning to move physicians from salary arrangements to productivity-based payment. Although this change is still too new to assess its impact, it marks the implementation of an important step to align physicians' financial interests with those of the hospital. However, some respondents expect this change to result in a significant decline in physicians' income in the short term. Physicians' response to these changes and their implications for hospital integration efforts remain to be seen.

Hospitals have also initiated a variety of care management programs, in contrast to two years ago, when little such activity was evident. In addition, these programs are notable for their efforts to improve care within the hospital and beyond the hospital walls.

For example, GHS has implemented a knee and hip replacement program that aims to reduce length of stay and improve overall recovery and functioning. Spartanburg Regional has implemented a program for patients with congestive heart failure, where nurses initiate contact with discharged patients to monitor and follow up on their chronic conditions. Readmissions have been lowered as a result.

But because they have not been accompanied by new financial arrangements, hospitals' continued efforts to improve care delivery have been hampered. In fact, with per diem reimbursement by health plans, hospitals that implement programs to reduce readmission rates and length of stay achieve significant cost savings for health plans—but they also substantially reduce the hospitals' own inpatient revenue.

Spartanburg Regional, for example, has tried to use these cost savings from quality improvement programs to negotiate better payment rates from plans, but has had limited success. Given the potential revenue loss, it is not known whether local hospitals will continue to pursue quality initiatives under current market conditions, or whether they will succeed in securing contracts that allow them to benefit financially from these activities.

Local Safety Net Improves, but Barriers Remain

While providers and social service groups noted serious gaps in the safety net in 1997, there appeared to be little public concern in the Greenville market about care for the poor. With no public hospital in the area, local hospital systems and community clinics acted as the major providers of indigent care, and their capacity was severely limited. Lack of public transportation—eliminated in early 1997 due to Greenville County's budget shortfalls—has exacerbated access problems. Meanwhile, Medicaid patients reportedly had difficulty getting appointments with private physicians, particularly pediatricians and primary care providers.

During the past two years, attention to the local safety net has heightened, and resources for meeting the needs of the poor have increased substantially. A community health assessment sponsored by the United Way brought to light the severity of Greenville's safety net problem and, according to market respondents, was an important catalyst for change. In addition, GHS has made significant new investments in care for the poor as it sought to improve its public image after the failed AGS merger. Finally, concerns about inappropriate emergency room utilization motivated both GHS and St. Francis to pledge funds to community clinics to bolster the local safety net.

As a result of these and other investments, two major safety net providers—the Greenville Community Health Center and the Greenville County Free Clinic—have been strengthened considerably. Both clinics have relocated to renovated facilities with expanded capacity and hours of operation. The Free Clinic also has added specialty services, such as ophthalmology and obstetrics-gynecology, and has opened a dental clinic. With more volunteer clinical staff, it aims to increase patient visits by 20 percent in 1999. The Greenville Community Health Center reports that it has already seen increases in its patient load.

Hospital systems in Spartanburg and Anderson counties have also taken steps to improve access for the uninsured. Spartanburg Regional recently opened a primary care clinic in a lower-income area of the county and relocated a number of its obstetrics-gynecology and primary care clinics to more accessible locations. Anderson Area Medical Center has expanded its community health service network and implemented a telephone triage program.

Access to care for Medicaid-eligible children also appears to have improved. Under an enhanced primary care case management (PCCM) program implemented by the state in lieu of mandating enrollment in HMOs, the state streamlined enrollment and coordination of care, and increased payments for primary care physicians leading to higher participation rates.

In addition, under a new state program, Partners for Healthy Children, children's eligibility for Medicaid has been extended to 150 percent of the federal poverty level for children up to age 18. By November 1998, the state had increased enrollment under the expanded program by 56,000 (its target is 75,000), thanks to successful outreach activities by local public health departments and higher payments for participating physicians.

Persistent obstacles to Medicaid recipients' enrollment in HMOs, however, make it unlikely that the state's plans for mandatory HMO enrollment will move forward. Although the state won federal approval in 1994 to require Medicaid recipients to enroll in HMOs, it never implemented the program because of concerns about plan capacity and limited cost savings potential. Medicaid recipients can enroll in HMOs on a voluntary basis, but few Greenville-area beneficiaries opt for this choice because the enrollment process is reportedly cumbersome, and many physicians prefer the payment arrangements under PCCM.

Despite many improvements in the local safety net, barriers to access remain. It appears that demand for care among the poor continues to outstrip available capacity, as evidenced by long waits to see safety net providers. Lack of public transportation remains a major access barrier for low-income residents. Greenville Community Health Center, for example, discontinued its expanded Saturday evening programs reportedly due in part to residents' difficulty getting to the clinic.

Issues to Track

Other than some improvements to the safety net, there has been less change in the Greenville market over the past two years than was anticipated. Hospital competition continues to thrive in light of the failed AGS merger, with an increasing focus on an area of rapid economic growth between Greenville and Spartanburg. HMO enrollment remains minimal, and fee-for-service payment continues to prevail. Nonetheless, hospitals have established productivity-based payment for physicians and continue their efforts to improve clinical care delivery.

Key issues to track in Greenville include the following:

- How will hospital competition across the market and within submarkets evolve? What impact will anticipated ownership change and new opportunities for joint ventures have on local market dynamics?
- Will hospital systems succeed in negotiating contracts that allow them to benefit financially from their efforts to integrate physician practices and improve clinical care management?
- What effect will productivity-based compensation have on physicians and their relationships with hospitals?
- What impact will recent capital improvements to the safety net and improvements to Medicaid have on access to care for the poor?

Consolidation Continues, Financial Pressures Mount

At the time of HSC's 1997 site visit, hospitals in northern New Jersey had recently undergone extensive consolidation in response to hospital rate deregulation and expected managed care growth. The subsequent closure of one inner city hospital triggered concerns that services would become concentrated in the suburbs and access to care in the inner city would deteriorate. Since then, hospital merger activity has slowed. Dire predictions concerning access to care in the inner city and the viability of the local safety net have not materialized, although some downsizing has occurred. Meanwhile, health plan consolidation has proceeded swiftly due to national and local mergers.

Other key developments since 1997 include:

- Two health plans folded amid allegations of unsound financial deals, mismanagement and inadequate state oversight, causing disruption for providers and consumers.
- hospitals and many health plans have struggled with poor financial performance.
- Efforts to establish physician-hospital contracting entities and expand risk arrangements have foundered.

Diverse Market with Local and Regional Influences

The northern New Jersey market, as defined by the Newark PMSA, spans a diverse area, including a number of inner cities, affluent suburbs and

NORTHERN NEW JERSEY DEMOGRAPHICS

	Northern New Jersey	Metropolitan areas above 200,000 population
Population, 1997[1]	1,943,494	
Population Change, 1990-1997[1]	1.4%	6.7%
Median Income[2]	$29,355	$26,646
Persons Living in Poverty[2]	10%	15%
Persons Age 65 or Older[2]	14%	12%
Persons with No Health Insurance[2]	9.8%	14%

Sources: 1. U.S. Census, 1997; 2. Household Survey, Community Tracking Study, 1996-1997

rural communities. It is noted for its high concentration of both wealth and poverty and significant ethnic and racial disparities. Health status is also highly variable; rates of AIDS and substance abuse in the city of Newark are among the nation's highest.

The area's urban-suburban split segments the hospital market, with some systems squarely anchored in the suburbs and others operating almost entirely in the inner cities. In contrast, health plans typically operate on a statewide or regional basis, with broad provider networks to accommodate the area's large employers and many commuters to and from nearby New York, Pennsylvania and Delaware. With unemployment at only 4.8 percent, employers offer generous, nonrestrictive health benefits to attract workers. Health maintenance organization (HMO) penetration remains low (just 24 percent, compared with an average of 34 percent for metropolitan areas), and organized activity by purchasers is minimal.

State policy has played an important role in shaping the health care market in northern New Jersey, although its focus has changed in recent years. In the early 1990s, the state began to deregulate the hospital industry. Hospital rate setting was abolished, a process for relaxing and streamlining certificate of need (CON) regulations was initiated and the state program for reimbursing hospitals for charity care was restructured and scaled back. Since then, the state has continued efforts to expand access to insurance, building on small-group and individual insurance market reforms passed in 1992. Premium subsidies for the working poor were enacted in 1995, and a new children's health insurance program, NJKidCare, was established in April 1998.

Like many other states, New Jersey has turned its attention to regulating managed care and has been particularly aggressive in this regard. The broad-ranging Health Care Quality Act (HCQA), signed into law in August

1997, contains provisions for consumer protections and a health plan report card that documents patient satisfaction and health plan performance on a variety of clinical measures.

Turmoil in the Health Plan Market

The collapse of two health plans has shaken the northern New Jersey market. Questionable financial arrangements and poor management allegedly led to the failures of both HIP of New Jersey, a prominent group-model HMO, and American Preferred Provider Plan (APPP), a relatively new plan that mainly served the Medicaid market.

Following several years of heavy losses, HIP was in desperate financial shape by 1997. HIP sold its physician practices and clinics to PHP Healthcare, a Virginia-based national health care management company, and subcontracted with PHP to provide physician services to its enrollees. The state approved the deal, even though PHP was heavily in debt and was operating at a loss. Although PHP's financial condition worsened and became more visible, the state contended that it had little regulatory authority to intervene because the arrangement was a subcontract and PHP was based outside of the state. When PHP subsequently went bankrupt, the state took over HIP's operations and ultimately moved to dissolve it.

The demise of APPP began when its owner diverted plan funds to two affiliated businesses that subsequently defaulted on the loans. When APPP's net worth fell below state solvency requirements, the state assumed control of the health plan and filed for bankruptcy on its behalf.

After each collapse, the state took measures to ensure continuity of care and facilitate the transfer of enrollees to other plans. These actions appear to have been largely successful. In the case of APPP, the state was able to transfer all 32,000 Medicaid enrollees to another plan. HIP's liquidation caused greater displacement, requiring more than 190,000 consumers— including an estimated 25,000 Medicaid beneficiaries—to find a new health plan. The state mandated a 30-day open enrollment period during which all plans were required to offer coverage at their usual rates. However, these rates were frequently higher than what consumers had paid before, and by the last week of the open enrollment period, an estimated 30,000 HIP members had not selected another plan. In addition, the closure of HIP's clinics resulted in physician and staff layoffs and some inherent disruptions in continuity of care.

The plans' failures also have had serious financial repercussions for providers, with estimates of debts of $80-$120 million in the case of HIP and more than $37 million in the case of APPP. Under recent settlements, hospitals and physicians will receive 30 cents on the dollar for all unpaid HIP claims for services prior to the state takeover and 20 to 23 cents on the dollar for unpaid APPP claims that preceded its takeover.

The collapse of HIP and APPP has raised concerns about the state's regulatory role. Health plan solvency requirements were raised in 1997, but the state is now taking steps to increase its regulatory oversight to prevent similar failures. In addition, legislative proposals, backed by the governor, would create a guaranty fund to help bail out financially troubled plans and to ensure provider payment in the event of a future crisis. Health plans would be required to contribute to this fund, though the New Jersey Association of Health Plans is vigorously opposing the idea, arguing that it constitutes a tax and would increase premiums.

Consolidation and Financial Woes

Rapid consolidation among hospitals was observed during HSC's 1997 site visit, and today this trend is seen most strikingly among health plans. Much of this is attributed to mergers among national plans, although the local Blue Cross Blue Shield plan's aggressive acquisition strategy also has played a role.

The most conspicuous and widely noted consolidation has been led by Aetna Inc., which, with more than one-third of HMO enrollees in northern New Jersey, is the largest HMO in the area. Its market share has grown substantially as a result of its 1997 merger with U.S. Healthcare and its subsequent acquisition of NYLCare in 1998. It stands to increase its market power even more with the recent federal approval of its acquisition of Prudential. Some providers and consumer groups fear that the resulting entity will command tremendous market leverage, reducing payments to providers, raising premiums and diminishing choice.

Meanwhile, Blue Cross Blue Shield of New Jersey has sought to reposition itself after state regulators blocked its proposed merger with Anthem, Inc., a multiregional Blues plan. Among other changes, the plan recently changed its name to Horizon Blue Cross Blue Shield of New Jersey to facilitate its entry into surrounding markets in Delaware and New York under the name "Horizon." This allows it to distinguish itself from other Blues plans that are licensed to sell branded products in those regions.

In general, health plans in this market, like their counterparts nationally, have confronted diminishing profit margins in recent years. After several years of holding down premiums to expand market share, plans are seeking increases of 10 percent or more in contracts negotiated in 1999.

In the hospital sector, the merger frenzy appears to have dissipated. In 1997, three major consolidations were underway, largely in response to regulatory change and expected managed care growth. Since then, these systems have continued to reconfigure through additional mergers or merger attempts; in one case, an existing partnership dissolved.

- St. Barnabas Health System, formed in 1995-1996, now includes 11 hospitals, five in northern New Jersey, and is the largest health care system in the state. The Clara Maass Medical Center recently joined the system, adding another 600 beds.
- Atlantic Health System, formed in 1996, consists of four community hospitals in the area. The system pursued a merger with the Robert Wood Johnson Health System, an eight-hospital system in New Brunswick, that would have given it more beds than St. Barnabas, but the deal came apart in early 1999 because of discrepancies over control and differences in mission.
- Finally, Via Caritas, a three-hospital Catholic system, formed in 1997, with plans to merge with the five-hospital Cathedral Healthcare System to create a unified local Catholic system. However, Cathedral opted to remain independent, arguing that it had little to gain from joining a larger system. Hospitals participating in Via Caritas began to think similarly, and the system dissolved in early 1999.

In a worsening financial environment, the two remaining merged systems, St. Barnabas and Atlantic, have struggled with poor financial performance. Although both systems have made strides toward administrative consolidation, there has been little consolidation of clinical services or capacity. Investments in infrastructure to coordinate functions at the system level also have exacted a cost. Moreover, the systems' financial performance has been strained by assuming the debt load and excess capacity of financially weak hospitals.

Statewide, hospitals' financial health has been eroding. According to the New Jersey Hospital Association, operating margins have decreased from 1.4 percent in 1996 to -1.3 percent in 1998. Hospitals attribute this decline to a variety of factors, including shortfalls in charity care funding from the state, financial repercussions of health plan failures and continuing payer demand for discounts. The federal Balanced Budget Act (BBA) of 1997 also has played a role, and downward pressure on hospital revenue is expected to intensify as the Act's remaining provisions are implemented. Hospitals have pressed the state for relief through increased charity care funding and stricter oversight of health plans to ensure timely and adequate payment. The state recently established a task force to determine other measures that may be necessary to strengthen hospitals' financial status.

Physician-Hospital Contracting Entities Off to Slow Start

One of the major objectives of the hospital systems formed in the past few years was to improve their bargaining position for managed care contracts. To this end, St. Barnabas and Atlantic each pursued strategies to coordinate contracting across the systems' hospitals and affiliated physicians. While each appears to have produced modest gains for the hospital partners, both faced setbacks to their physician integration efforts and have begun to revamp their strategies accordingly.

In January 1997, Atlantic launched a large-scale management services organization (MSO), Health Resource Partners (HRP), to handle managed care risk contracting for nearly 800 affiliated physicians across the four-hospital system. Atlantic invested $12 million in setting up HRP and building the infrastructure necessary to manage risk. However, it was unsuccessful in negotiating acceptable contract terms with plans because of plans' reluctance to delegate responsibility for clinical care management along with financial risk. The hospital system now has scaled back HRP to provide services for a physician organization associated with just one hospital.

St. Barnabas originally sought to build its network by purchasing physician practices, but, consistent with national trends, it has moved away from this strategy, which yielded fewer benefits than expected. It is currently developing the St. Barnabas Physician Partnership, a super physician-hospital organization (PHO), to coordinate contracting across all of the system's hospitals and affiliated physicians. At the time of the 1999 site visit, several hundred physicians had submitted applications to join, and the system is targeting more than 4,000 physicians. The partnership has been selected for a Medicare demonstration project to pilot the use of global payment at three hospitals, giving it an important large initial contract. Market observers note that this contract may help St. Barnabas's PHO to secure the scale needed to change the dynamics of local managed care contract negotiations.

Aside from these initiatives, physician organization remains quite limited in northern New Jersey. Most physicians continue to practice in solo or small-group practices. While there are many PHOs at local hospitals, they do not require physician exclusivity, so they wield little market power.

Safety Net Providers Adapt to Changing Environment

In 1997, many respondents reported that the northern New Jersey safety net was in peril, largely because of state policy changes with regard to deregulation of hospital rates and the adoption of mandatory Medicaid managed care. Both were expected to exert downward pressure on hospital payment, which many feared would threaten the financial viability of inner city hospitals in particular and diminish access to services for people living in urban areas.

Since then, providers' financial environment overall has worsened, and there has been some downsizing among safety net providers. However, the safety net, by and large, has not deteriorated to the extent anticipated, though serious financial pressures remain.

The state scaled back funding for charity care with the implementation of hospital rate deregulation in 1992, resulting in a dramatic drop from $700 million that year to $500 million in 1993. Funding levels continued to decline steadily for several years, reaching a low of $300 million in 1997. In 1998 and 1999, however, the state increased charity care funding to $320 million annually. The state also increased funding under the Hospital Relief Fund, which targets hospitals with a disproportionate share of high-cost cases, such as HIV/AIDS, tuberculosis and complex neonatal care. An additional $58 million was allocated under this fund in 1998, bringing it up to $183 million in total.

Recent increases in public subsidies for charity care have helped hospitals to hold their ground and have especially benefited inner city hospitals, where much of this care is concentrated. Nevertheless, hospitals' provision of charity care continues to exceed state funding, and inner city hospitals in particular continue to shoulder significant financial burdens related to un-compensated care.

Some inner city hospitals have pursued strategies that appear to have helped mitigate this financial pressure. For instance, Newark Beth Israel, an inner city tertiary care provider now part of the St. Barnabas system, appears to have been bolstered by its affiliation with financially stronger hospitals. Others have taken advantage of NJKidCare to secure reimbursement for previously uninsured patients. For example, one major local safety net provider, University Health System, noted its efforts to enroll eligible children on site to capture this revenue. Overall, however, slow enrollment in NJKidCare has limited the gains from this program.

Providers also have had to adapt to mandatory Medicaid managed care, which has been phased in rapidly since it was launched in 1995. The program now covers 95 percent of Medicaid beneficiaries eligible through the state's welfare program and is generating an estimated savings of $400 million a year. Moreover, the low auto-assignment rate relative to other states is considered by many to be a marker of the program's success in minimizing the potential negative impact on enrollees.

However, Medicaid managed care has produced financial strain for some safety net providers, particularly as the number of uninsured reportedly is growing. Community health centers (CHCs) report declines in revenue, largely due to reduced payment under capitation and reported increases in uncompensated care. As a result, several CHCs have closed sites, reduced hours and staff and scaled back outreach and education programs.

Issues to Track

The northern New Jersey health care market continues to experience significant change. While consolidation continues in both sectors, albeit more slowly for hospitals, the financial performance of hospitals and many health plans has worsened considerably. Hospitals are seeking additional state funding for some relief, while plans are looking to employers to increase premiums and, in some cases, relying on state bailouts. Meanwhile, local physicians, still largely unorganized, have secured little bargaining power in the market. At the same time, the safety net did not deteriorate as feared two years ago but remains financially strained.

As the market continues to change, several key issues warrant tracking:

- What impact will consolidation among health plans have on premiums, provider reimbursement and the nature of competition among plans and providers in the local market?
- How will the state's regulatory role evolve in terms of overseeing the financial solvency of health plans?
- Will the financial condition of hospitals stabilize? Will hospital systems move toward greater consolidation of clinical services and capacity? Will more mergers come apart?
- Will PHOs become more successful in securing risk contracts in the local market? Will greater physician organization emerge?
- Will safety net providers continue to remain viable? How will their continuing survival strategies affect the populations they serve?

Comparison of Communities HSC Tracks

The Community Tracking Study, the major effort of HSC, tracks changes in the health system in 60 sites that are representative of the nation. Every two years HSC conducts surveys in all 60 communities and site visits in the 12 communities, data from which are shown in the following tables.

GATEKEEPING AND COMPENSATION

	Insured Persons Covered Under Gatekeeping Arrangements	Physicians Receiving Capitation for At Least Some of Their Patients
Boston, MA	62 %+	61 %
Cleveland, OH	41 %+	63 %+
Greenville, SC	31 %+	43 %+
Indianapolis, IN	41 %+	67 %+
Lansing, MI	48 %	59 %
Little Rock, AR	50 %	44 %+
Miami, FL	52 %	60 %
Northern New Jersey	45 %	51 %
Orange County, CA	52 %+	72 %+
Phoenix, AZ	54 %+	59 %
Seattle, WA	43 %	73 %+
Syracuse, NY	35 %+	41 %+
Metropolitan Areas	46 %	56 %

Source: Community Tracking Study Physician Survey, 1996–1997
Note: The margin of error is ±3 percent to ±9 percent.
+ Site value is significantly different from the mean for metropolitan areas with over 200,000 population.

CONSUMER PERCEPTIONS OF ACCESS TO CARE

	Families Satisfied with the Health Care Received in the Last 12 Months	Patients Agreeing That Their Doctor Might Not Refer Them to a Specialist When Needed
Boston, MA	90 %	12 %+
Cleveland, OH	88 %	15 %
Greenville, SC	90 %	16 %
Indianapolis, IN	90 %	13 %
Lansing, MI	91 %	11 %+
Little Rock, AR	88 %	17 %
Miami, FL	84 %+	22 %+
Northern New Jersey	87 %	14 %
Orange County, CA	87 %	20 %+
Phoenix, AZ	87 %	18 %
Seattle, WA	89 %	13 %+
Syracuse, NY	92 %+	12 %+
Metropolitan Areas	88 %	16 %

Source: Community Tracking Study Household Survey, 1996–1997
Note: The margin of error is ±2 percent to ±5 percent.
+ Site value is significantly different from the mean for metropolitan areas with over 200,000 population.

PHYSICIAN PERCEPTIONS OF ACCESS TO CARE

	Physicians Not Agreeing That it is Possible to Provide High-Quality Care to All of Their Patients	Primary Care Physicians Reporting That They Cannot Always or Almost Always Obtain Referrals to High-Quality Specialists When Medically Necessary
Boston, MA	23 %	12 %+
Cleveland, OH	21 %	14 %+
Greenville, SC	19 %+	14 %+
Indianapolis, IN	24 %	6 %+
Lansing, MI	18 %+	19 %
Little Rock, AR	21 %	17 %
Miami, FL	30 %	31 %+
Northern New Jersey	29 %	31 %+
Orange County, CA	31 %	26 %
Phoenix, AZ	30 %	23 %

(continued on facing page)

	Physicians Not Agreeing That it is Possible to Provide High-Quality Care to All of Their Patients	*Primary Care Physicians Reporting That They Cannot Always or Almost Always Obtain Referrals to High-Quality Specialists When Medically Necessary*
Seattle, WA	25 %	15 %+
Syracuse, NY	18 %+	13 %+
Metropolitan Areas	25 %	20 %+

Source: Community Tracking Study Physician Survey, 1996–1997
Note: The margin of error is ±3 percent to ±9 percent.
+ Site value is significantly different from the mean for metropolitan areas with over 200,000 population.

EMPLOYERS AND HEALTH INSURANCE *(based on preliminary data)*

	Employers Offering Health Insurance	*Average Monthly Premium for Employer-Sponsored Health Insurance*
Boston, MA	54 %	$198
Cleveland, OH	61 %	$164
Greenville, SC	44 %	$152
Indianapolis, IN	53 %	$178
Lansing, MI	56 %	$184
Little Rock, AR	52 %	$159
Miami, FL	40 %	$160
Northern New Jersey	47 %	$197
Orange County, CA	47 %	$156
Phoenix, AZ	48 %	$158
Seattle, WA	52 %	$184
Syracuse, NY	50 %	$163
United States	50 %	$171

Source: The Robert Wood Johnson Foundation Employer Health Insurance Survey, 1997
Note: The margin of error is ±4 percent to ±8 percent.

References

Anders, G., and L. McGinley. 1998. "Actuarial Firm Helps Decide Just How Long You Spend in Hospital." *Wall Street Journal* (June 15): A1, A16.

APM/ University Health System Consortium. 1995. "How Markets Evolve." *Hospitals & Health Networks* 69 (5): 60.

Bamezai, A., J. Zwanziger, G. A. Melnick, and J. M. Mann. 1999. "Price Competition and Hospital Cost Growth in the United States (1989-1994)." *Health Economics* 8 (3): 233–243.

Berlin, I. 1993. *The Hedgehog and the Fox.* Chicago: Elephant Paperbacks.

Bindman, A. B., K. Grumbach, S. Bernheim, K. Vranizan, M. Cousineau. 2000. "Medicaid Managed Care's Impact on Safety-Net Clinics in California." *Health Affairs* 19 (1): 194–202.

Blendon, R. J, M. Brodie, J. M. Benson, D. E. Altman, L. Levitt, T. Hoff, and L. Hugick. 1998. "Understanding the Managed Care Backlash." *Health Affairs* 17 (4): 80–94.

Blue Cross and Blue Shield Association. 2001. "Our History: About the Blue Cross and Blue Shield Association." [Online information; retrieved 2/15/01]. www.bcbs.com/whoweare/history.html.

Bodenheimer, T. 1999. "The American Health Care System-Physicians and The Changing Medical Marketplace." *The New England Journal of Medicine* 340 (7): 584–588.

Bogue, R. J., S. M. Shortell, M. Sohn, L. Manheim, G. Bazzoli, and C. Chan. 1995. "Hospital Reorganization After Merger." *Medical Care* 33 (7): 676–686.

Brett, A. 1997. "Relationships Between Primary Care Physicians and Consultants in Managed Care." *The Journal of Clinical Ethics* 8 (1): 60–65.

Brooks, J. M., A. Dor, and H. S. Wong. 1997. "Hospital-Insurer Bargaining: An Empirical Investigation of Appendectomy Pricing." *Journal of Health Economics* 16 (4): 417–434.

Brown, L. D. 1983. *Politics and Health Care Organization HMOs as Federal Policy.* Washington, DC: Brookings Institution.

—. 1997. "The Metamorphosis: Conversion in Historical Context." *Bulletin of the New York Academy of Medicine* 74 (2): 238–47.

Cain Brothers. 1997. *The Blue Cross and Blue Shield Plans: Coping With Change, Regaining Momentum, Providing Leadership.* New York: Cain Brothers.

Center for Studying Health System Change. 1999. *Results From Tracking 12 Communities, 1997-1999. Compilation of Round Two Site Visits.* Washington, DC: Center for Studying Health System Change.

Christianson, J. 1998. "The Role of Employers in Community Health Care Systems." *Health Affairs* 17 (4): 158–64.

Community Catalyst. 1999. "New England's Blue Cross Blue Shield Shake-Out: A Case Study in Consumer Activism." *States of Health* 9 (4).

Consumers Union. 2000a. "Conversion and Preservation of Charitable Assets of Blue Cross and Blue Shield Plans: How States Have Protected or Failed to Protect the Public Interest." [Online article; retrieved 11/15/00]. www.consumersunion.org/health/bcbswc600.htm.

—. 2000b. "Consumer Groups Call on Washington Officials to Protect Public's Investment in Blue Cross and Blue Shield." [Online Press Release; retrieved 11/15/00]. www.consumersunion.org/health/washwc900.htm.

Corrigan, J. M., J. S. Eden, M. R. Gold, and J. D. Pickreign. 1997. "Trends Toward a National Health Care Marketplace." *Inquiry* 34 (1): 11–28.

Cunningham, R., and R. M. Cunningham. 1997. *The Blues: A History of the Blue Cross and Blue Shield System.* DeKalb, IL: Northern Illinois University Press.

Cunningham, P. J. 1999. "Pressures on the Safety Net: Differences in Access to Care for Uninsured Persons by the Level of Managed Care Penetration and Uninsurance Rate in a Community." *Health Services Research* 34 (1, Part 2): 255–70.

Cunningham, P. J., J. M. Grossman, R. F. St. Peter, and C. S. Lesser. 1999. "Managed Care and Physicians' Provision of Charity Care." *Journal of the American Medical Association* 281 (12): 1087–92.

Defino, T. 1994. "Capitating Specialty Care." *HMO Magazine* (July/August): 73–76.

Dickens, C. 1998 edition. *Hard Times.* New York: Oxford University Press.

Dranove, D., and R. Ludwick, 1999. "Competition and Pricing by Nonprofit Hospitals: A Reassessment of Lynk's Analysis." *Journal of Health Economics* 18 (1): 87–98.

Enthoven, A. C., and S. J. Singer, 1998. "The Managed Care Backlash and the Task Force in California." *Health Affairs* 17 (4): 95–110.

Ferreter, M. 2000. "Taking Their Cut." *Modern Physician* (January): 40–43.

Forgione, D. A. 1999. "Those Conversion Blues." *Journal of Healthcare Finance* 25 (4): 38–46.

Fossett, J. W. et al. 1999. *Managing Accountability in Medicaid Managed Care: The Politics of Public Management.* Albany, NY: Nelson A. Rockefeller Institute of Government.

Foubister, V. 1999. "Specialty Group's Pick-Up Speed." *American Medical News* (August 16): 1–6.

Frech, H. E. 1996. *Competition and Monopoly in Medical Care.* Washington, DC: The AEI Press.

Friedman, E. 1998. "What Price Survival? The Future of Blue Cross and Blue Shield." *Journal of the American Medical Association* 279 (23): 1863–9.

Gabel, J. 1997. "Ten Ways HMOs Have Changed During the 1990s." *Health Affairs* 16 (3): 134–45.

Ginsburg, P. B., and C. S. Lesser. 1999. "The View from Communities." *Journal of Health Politics, Policy and Law* 24 (5): 1005–1013.

Ginsburg, P., P. Kemper, L. Kohn, and R. Baxter. 2000. "The Community Tracking Study Analyses of Market Change: Introduction and Methods." *Health Services Research* 35 (1): 7–16.

Glied, S. 2000. "Managed Care." In *Handbook of Health Economics, edited by* A.J. Culyer and J. P. Newhouse, 708–753. Elsevier Science.

Gold, M. 1999. "Making Medicaid Managed Care Research Relevant." *Health Services Research* 33 (6): 1639–1650.

Grogan, C. M, and M. K. Gusmano. 1999. "State Report: How are Safety-Net Providers Faring Under Medicaid Managed Care?" *Health Affairs* 18 (2): 233–237.

Grossman, J. 2000. "Health Plan Competition in Local Markets." *Health Services Research* 35 (1): 17–36.

Guglielmo, W. 1996. "How to Avoid Deselection." *Medical Economics* (April 15): 149–151, 154.

Harris, G., M. Ripperger, and H. Hom. 2000. "Managed Care at the Crossroads." *Health Affairs* 19 (1): 157–163.

Holahan, J., S. Zuckerman, A. Evans, and S. Rangarajan. 1998. "Medicaid Managed Care in Thirteen States." *Health Affairs* 17 (3): 43–63.

—. 1999. "Medicaid Payment Methods and Capitation Rates: Results of a National Survey." Occasional Paper, no. 26. Washington, DC: Urban Institute.

Iglehart, J. 1994. "Physicians and the Growth of Managed Care." *The New England Journal of Medicine* 331 (17): 1167–1171.

InterStudy Publications. 2000. *The InterStudy Competitive Edge 10.2, Part II: HMO Industry Report.* St. Paul, MN: InterStudy Publications.

Irving Levin Associates. 1999. *The Hospital Acquisition Report*. New Canaan, CT: Irving Levin Associates, Inc.

Jacobs, L. R., and R. Y. Shapiro. 1999. "The American Public's Pragmatic Liberalism Meets its Philosophical Conservatism." *Journal of Health Politics, Policy and Law* 24 (5): 1021–1031.

Jaklevic, M. 1999. "Remembering the Specialists." *Modern Healthcare* 29 (17): 35–36, 38.

Jarillo, J., and J. Ricart. 1987. "Sustaining Networks." *Interfaces* 17 (5): 82–91.

Jarillo, J. 1988. "On Strategic Networking." *Strategic Management Journal* 9: 31–41.

Jensen, G., M. Morrisey, S. Gaffney, and D. Lipton. 1997. "The New Dominance of Managed Care: Insurance Trends in the 1990s." *Health Affairs* 16 (1): 125–36.

Journal of Health Politics, Policy and Law. 1999. "Special Issue: The Managed Care Backlash." 24 (October): 873–1218.

Kaiser Commission on the Future of Medicaid. 1995. *Medicaid and Managed Care: Lessons from the Literature*. Washington: DC: Kaiser Commission.

Katz, A. 2000. Personal Communication.

Keeler, E. B., G. Melnick, and J. Zwanziger. 1999. "The Changing Effects of Competition on Non-Profit and For-Profit Hospital Pricing Behavior." *Journal of Health Economics* 18 (1): 69–86.

Kemper, P., D. Blumenthal, J. Corrigan, P. Cunningham, S. Felt, J. Grossman, L. Kohn, C. Metcalf, R. St. Peter, R. Strouse, and P. Ginsburg. 1996. "The Design of the Community Tracking Study: A Longitudinal Study of Health System Change and Its Effects on People." *Inquiry* 33 (2): 195–206.

Kohn, L. T., P. Kemper, R. J. Baxter, R. L. Feldman, and P. B. Ginsburg (eds). 1997. *Health System Change in Twelve Communities*. Washington, DC: Center for Studying Health System Change.

Kohn, L. 2000. "Organizing and Managing Care in a Changing Health System." *Health Services Research* 35 (1): 37–52.

Lesser, C. S., and P. B. Ginsburg. 2000. "Update on the Nation's Health Care System: 1997-1999." *Health Affairs* 19 (6): 206–16.

Lillie-Blanton, M., and B. Lyons. 1998. "Medicaid and Low-Income Populations: Recent State Experience." *Health Affairs* 17 (May/June): 238–247.

Lipson, D. J. 1997. "Medicaid Managed Care and Community Providers: New Partnerships." *Health Affairs* 16 (4): 91–107.

Marsteller, J. A., and R. R. Bovberg. 1999. "Federalism and Patient Protection Changing Roles for State and Federal Government." Occasional Paper, no. 28. Washington, DC: Urban Institute.

McCall, N. 1997. "Lessons from Arizona's Medicaid Managed Care Program." *Health Affairs* 16 (4): 194–199.

McCue, M. J., R. E. Hurley, D. A. Draper, and M. Jurgensen. 1999. "Reversal of Fortune: Commercial HMOs in the Medicaid Market." *Health Affairs* 18 (1): 223–230.

Melnick, G.A., J. Zwanziger, A. Bamezai, and R. Pattison. 1992. "The Effects of Market Structure and Bargaining Position on Hospital Prices." *Journal of Health Economics* 11 (3): 217–233.

Montague, J. 1996. "Specialists at the Gate." *Hospital & Health Networks* 70 (16): 38.

Moran, M. 1999. *Governing the Health Care State: A Comparative Study of the United Kingdom, the United States and Germany.* Manchester, UK: Manchester University Press.

Newark Star-Ledger Archive. 1998. "Series: A Failed Union; The HIP-PHP Debacle." *Newark Star-Ledger Archive* (December 12).

New York Times. 1999. "Feeling the Push of Managed Care." *New York Times* (February 12): B1, B6.

Oster, S. 1999. *Modern Competitive Analysis,* 3rd edition. New York: Oxford University Press.

Peterson, M. A. 1999. "Introduction: Politics, Misperception, or Apropos?" *Journal of Health Politics, Policy and Law* 24 (October): 873–886.

Porter, M. 1998. "How Competitive Forces Shape Strategy." In *On Competition.* Boston: Harvard Business Review School Publishing.

Robinson, J., and L. Casalino. 1995. "Growth of Medical Groups Paid Through Capitation in California." *New England Journal of Medicine* 333 (25): 1684–1687.

Robinson, J. 1999. "The Future of Managed Care Organization." *Health Affairs* 18(12): 7–24.

Robinson, J. C. 2000. "Capital Finance and Ownership Conversions in Health Care." *Health Affairs* 19 (1): 56–71.

Rochefort, D. A. 1998. "The Role of Anecdotes in Regulating Managed Care." *Health Affairs* 17 (6): 142–149.

Rowland, D., and K. Hanson. 1996. "Medicaid: Moving to Managed Care." *Health Affairs* 15 (Fall): 150–152.

Simpson, J., and R. Shin. 1998. "Do Nonprofit Hospitals Exercise Market Power?" *International Journal of the Economics of Business* 5 (2): 141–158.

Simon, C., and P. Dorn. 1996. "Physician Earnings in a Changing Managed Care Environment." *Health Affairs* 15 (3): 124–133.

Sisk, J. 1998. "How Are Health Care Organizations Using Clinical Guidelines?" *Health Affairs* 17 (5): 91–109.

Solomon, L. 1998. "Rules of the Game: How Public Policy Affects Local Health Care Markets." *Health Affairs* 17 (4): 140–48.

Sparer, M. et al. 1996. "Managed Care and Low-Income Populations: A Case Study of Managed Care in California." Washington, DC: Mathematica Policy Research, Inc.

Sparer, M., and L. D. Brown. 1999. "Nothing Exceeds Like Success: Managed Care Comes to Medicaid in New York City." *Milbank Quarterly* 77 (2): 205–23, 174.

—. 2000. "Uneasy Alliances: Managed Care Plans Formed by Safety-Net

Providers." *Health Affairs* 19 (July/August): 23–35.

Trude, S., T. West, and S. McIntosh. 1999. *Competition Intensifies After Proposed Merger Fails: Community Report, Greenville, South Carolina*. Washington, DC: Center for Studying Health Systems Change.

U.S. Government Accounting Office. 1994. *Blue Cross and Blue Shield: Experiences of Weak Plans Underscore the Role of Effective State Oversight: Report to the Chairman, Permanent Subcommittee on Investigations, Committee on Governmental Affairs, U.S. Senate*. Washington, DC: U.S. GAO (GAO/HEHS 94–71).

Woolley, J. M. 1989. "The Competitive Effects of Horizontal Mergers in the Hospital Industry." *Journal of Health Economics* 8 (3): 271–291.

About The Center
for Studying Health
System Change

The Center for Studying Health System Change (HSC) is a nonpartisan policy research organization located in Washington, DC. Started in 1995, HSC is funded exclusively by The Robert Wood Johnson Foundation and is affiliated with Mathematica Policy Research, Inc.

HSC's mission is to provide objective and timely insights on changes in the nation's healthcare system to inform policymakers, thereby contributing to the formation of better healthcare policy.

HSC's research is grounded in the Community Tracking Study (CTS), a national study of health system change based on surveys and site visits. Under the CTS, HSC fields surveys of households, physicians, and employers every two years to gather perspectives about the ways that the health system is changing and the effects on consumers. In addition, site visits are conducted every two years to examine changes in the organization and financing of care and the changing nature of competition in local healthcare markets.

The CTS surveys are conducted in 60 communities that were randomly selected to be nationally representative, and the site visits are conducted in 12 of these communities.

HSC publications and public use files of the survey data are available on its web site at www.hschange.org.

About the Authors

PAUL B. GINSBURG, PH.D., is president of the Center for Studying Health System Change (HSC). Founded in 1995, HSC conducts a wide range of research focused on changes in healthcare financing and delivery in the United States. Prior to joining HSC, Dr. Ginsburg served as the founding executive director of the Physician Payment Review Commission (now the Medicare Payment Advisory Commission), which developed the Medicare physician payment reform proposal that was enacted by Congress in 1989 and has since been implemented. In addition, Dr. Ginsburg was a senior economist at RAND and served as deputy assistant director at the Congressional Budget Office. Before that, he served on the faculties of Duke University and Michigan State University. Dr. Ginsburg is a noted speaker and consultant on the changes taking place in the healthcare system. He served for two terms on the board of directors of the Association for Health Services Research and is a founding member of the National Academy of Social Insurance, where he chaired a panel on reforming the Medicare program. He earned his doctorate in economics from Harvard University.

CARA S. LESSER, M.P.P., is a health researcher at HSC and is responsible for overall management of HSC's Community Tracking Study's site visits in 12 communities and production of the *Community Reports*—HSC's related publication series. Ms. Lesser's current research projects include assessing how local health systems have changed over the past two years and the impact of hospital mergers on local markets. Prior to joining HSC, Ms. Lesser was at the Institute for Health Policy Studies at the University of California at San Francisco, where she conducted research on state health-reform initiatives. Ms. Lesser received a M.P.P. from the University of California at Berkeley.

Linda R. Brewster, M.B.A., is an independent consultant and has been providing research assistance to HSC in the area of how hospitals and physicians are affected by changes in the health system. In addition to assisting with the planning and design of the data-collection process, Ms. Brewster is involved in conducting the current round of site visits and is involved in research focusing on changes in hospitals' strategic behavior, particularly with respect to integrating physicians. Prior to her work at HSC, Ms. Brewster has held leadership positions within several hospital-sponsored physician integration organizations. She was also executive director of the Massachusetts Institute of Technology's Health Plan and Medical Department. Ms. Brewster received a M.B.A. from Harvard Graduate School of Business Administration.

Lawrence D. Brown, Ph.D., is a professor in the Division of Health Policy and Management at the Joseph L. Mailman School of Public Health of Columbia University. Before coming to Columbia in 1988, Dr. Brown was a senior fellow in the Brookings Institution's Governmental Studies Program and a professor at the University of Michigan's School of Public Health, where he directed the PEW Trust Health Policy Program. Dr. Brown is a member of the National Advisory Committees of The Robert Wood Johnson Foundation's Investigator's Program, its Urban Health Initiative Program, the United Hospital Fund's President Council, and the board of the Community Services Society. He is a research adviser to HSC. From 1984-1989, he was editor of the *Journal of Health Politics, Policy and Law*. Dr. Brown is the author of *Politics and Health Care Organization: HMOs as Federal Policy* (Brookings, 1983) and various monographs and articles. He writes on competitive and regulatory issues in health, on the politics of state and national strategies to achieve affordable universal coverage, and on the uses of policy analysis in the policy process. He received a Ph.D. in government from Harvard University.

Jon B. Christianson, Ph.D., is an economist with extensive research and teaching experience in the financing and delivery of medical care. He has written publications in the areas of managed care, rural healthcare, mental healthcare, and care process involvement. He has also collaborated with healthcare providers in a variety of practice settings to evaluate new treatment approaches. Currently, Dr. Christianson serves on the faculty of the Carlson School of Management at the University of

Minnesota, where he is the James A. Hamilton chair in Health Policy and Management. Dr. Christianson serves on a number of different editorial boards and scientific advisory panels, and he directs the Center for the Study of Healthcare Management in the Department of Healthcare Management at the Carlson School. He received his Ph.D. from the University of Wisconsin-Madison.

JOY GROSSMAN, PH.D., is associate director of HSC and oversees HSC's research and data-collection activities. Dr. Grossman's research focus is on competition in local healthcare markets and market variation in managed care. Before joining HSC, Dr. Grossman was a health policy analyst with the Prospective Payment Assessment Commission. In this position and in prior research positions at the University of California at San Francisco and Berkeley, she worked on a variety of issues related to hospital financing and competition. As an investment banker in New York, she arranged tax-exempt financing for nonprofit hospitals. Dr. Grossman earned a Ph.D. in economics from the University of California at Berkeley.

BRADLEY STRUNK is a health research analyst at HSC. Mr. Strunk's current research is focused on the managed care industry, the role of Blue Cross and Blue Shield Plans, and access to healthcare services among the U.S. population. He has also worked extensively on the site visit component of HSC's Community Tracking Study. Prior to joining HSC, Mr. Strunk worked at the Department of Public Health Sciences at the Wake Forest University School of Medicine, where he studied the implications of tobacco-reform efforts on rural tobacco farmers across the United States. Mr. Strunk received a bachelor's degree in economics from Wake Forest University.